The Nurses' Career Guide

The
Nurses'
Career Guide

*Discovering New Horizons
in Health Care*

Zardoya E. Eagles, R.N.

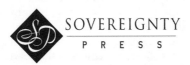

SOVEREIGNTY
PRESS

The Nurses' Career Guide: Discovering New Horizons In Health Care
© 1997 by Zardoya E. Eagles

Sovereignty Press
1241 Johnson Avenue, #353
San Luis Obispo, CA 93401

Manufactured in the United States of America
First printing February 1997
04 03 02 01 00 99 98 97   10 9 8 7 6 5 4 3 2 1

Illustrations by Jorel Williams, Minneapolis, Minnesota
Cover design © 1997 by Lightbourne Images, Ashland, Oregon
Editing & interior design by Sara Patton, Maui, Hawaii

Publisher's Cataloging in Publication
(Prepared by Quality Books Inc.)

Eagles, Zardoya E.
    The nurses' career guide : discovering new horizons in health care /
by Zardoya E. Eagles.
    p. cm.
    Includes bibliographical references and index.
    ISBN 0-9656025-8-3

    1. Nursing — Vocational guidance.   I. Title.

RT82.E34 1997   610.73'06'9
                                             QBI96-40844

Library of Congress Catalog Card Number: 96-93097

. . . .

This publication is designed to provide accurate, authoritative, and motivational information on the topic of career development. It is sold with the understanding that the publisher and author are not engaged in rendering career management advice or other professional career management services. If professional assistance is required, the services of an appropriate expert should be sought.

This book is dedicated to the hundreds of nurses who have approached me over the years, asking, "So, how did you get your job?"

May it serve as a springboard to a clearer understanding of how you can make your unique contribution to the profession of nursing.

Contents

Thank you to the following publishers, who generously gave permission to use quotations from their copyrighted works.

From *The New Mentors and Protégés* by Linda Phillips-Jones. Copyright 1993 by Linda Phillips-Jones. Used with permission of the Coalition of Counseling Centers, Grass Valley, California.

From *Getting Hired in the '90s* by Vicki Spina. Copyright 1995 by Vicki Spina. Used with permission of the publisher, Dearborn Financial Publishing, Inc., Chicago, Illinois. All rights reserved.

From *Living Without a Goal* by James Ogilvy. Copyright 1995 by James Ogilvy. Used with permission of Bantam Doubleday Dell Publishing Group, Inc., New York, New York.

Acknowledgments

Over the years, I've quickly glanced through the acknowledgments in many books, and stifled a yawn as I thought, "Come on, let's get on with it." I have a new appreciation for all of those kind words and thank-you's—an appreciation that comes from the heartfelt realization that there is *no way* this book would have been completed without the loving support of many people. They are all contributors to this project, and I simply can't publish this book without properly acknowledging them. So, if you're already yawning, just skip right to the introduction...

My many thanks to:

Marti Koch, for helping me turn a vague dissatisfaction with my job into a journey that led not only to my own future, but also to the production of this book;

Linda Phillips-Jones, for helping me understand the nature of mentoring partnerships, and *Rita Farnham,* for stepping into the role of mentor/advisor/clarifier/inspirer during the evolution of this book;

Jorel Williams, for creating illustrations that exactly capture the feeling and tone of this book, and being a great friend and source of support for many years;

Sara Patton, for using her fine editing and layout skills to "polish" the manuscript and make each word fall into its right place;

Shannon Bodie at Lightbourne Images, who seemed to "see" exactly what was in my mind and then beautifully create the images that made the cover come to life;

Linda Nicolson, Bonnie Thanos, Tammie Windish, Karen Williams, Rita Farnham, Karen Olson, and *Jennifer Tomberlin,* who provided peer review on the manuscript, offered valuable feedback and support, and helped me to create a book that speaks to a broader audience of nurses;

The many people who encouraged and supported me on this journey, especially *Dana Ott, Shari Collom,* and *Mark Wilson;*

My parents, *Bev and Jerry Stumpf,* and all my brothers and sisters: *Kathy, Barbara, Carol, Bob, Marilyn, Dick, Julie, Pat, Tom,* and *Teri,* for keeping the doorway to "home" open and never giving up on me;

Special thanks to my sister *Marilyn Bayerl,* her husband *Tim,* and children *Rhonda* and *Rob,* for providing me a haven on beautiful Lake Mary last summer; and to my sister *Teri Holgate,* who is always there with support and ideas and who spent days cross-checking the resource guide for this book;

Susan Pendergast, for her unremitting wisdom and support in helping me bring forth my beautiful offering, and for all the late-night phone calls (to calm nerves and quell waves of panic);

And finally, *Nadia K. Eagles,* my teacher and mentor, for helping me discover my unique contribution to the world . . . and then giving me the tools I need to *make* that contribution.

My life has been enriched by each of these remarkable people.

Just past the distant horizon lies the future...

And each step forward reveals another new expanse of future before you.

A never-ending life journey.

But when you follow your inner sense of knowing,

The journey becomes the joy.

The outcome becomes incidental.

And truth becomes your daily guide.

Introduction

New horizons in health care ... did you ever think you'd be looking at nursing from this perspective? Always seen as very practical and down-to-earth, members of the nursing profession are currently going through such tremendous change that we really *need* a bird's-eye view, a perspective from "above it all," to begin to sort out the tangle of feelings and realities that are affecting the daily choices that we have to make. This perspective, however, is not a given. It is *earned* by working to develop an understanding of ourselves, our role as nurses, and our individual hopes, dreams, and goals. It is earned by taking the risk to look at the entire truth—our own inner truth *and* the truth about what exists out in the world. Whether you are just starting out as a new graduate or you've been in nursing for 30 years, a solid foundation of self-understanding is essential. We each need to know what we truly want in order to visualize and create the future of our dreams.

This book is designed to provide you with practical insight and information to guide you through the process of planning your future in nursing. It is written based on my own personal journey through this terrain and includes years of research for classes I've taught on change management, burnout, and career development. It comes from the heart—and from a deep sense of knowing that nurses are some of the strongest, most capable people on this planet.

In the 15 years I've been in nursing, working first as a staff nurse in ICU/CCU, then in labor and delivery, and most recently as an educator and consultant, I have met nurses of all types. Especially in the past five years as a consultant, I have come into contact with thousands of nurses in hospitals all over the country (hundreds of them wanting to know how I got my job!). What I've found is a group of people with a nearly universal strength of character, vast creativity and resourcefulness, and the ability to coordinate many things at once and manage an absolute *bombardment* of changes every day. It was only after I went through an extensive career search and ended up working in the "business world" that I was able to see how *rare* these qualities are outside of the nursing profession.

Nurses are working very hard to continue providing quality care under sometimes adverse conditions. We carry on relentlessly, trying to stay ahead of the tides of change, often unaware of how valuable our skills really are. Many nurses express a desire to make a career change. Many new grads are struggling to find a place in health care. Unfortunately, few understand the types of opportunities that exist both within and outside the traditional role of hospital nursing—not to mention what it takes to find the way through the seemingly never-ending process of change to access those opportunities.

Now is the time to make friends with the change process. This book is a tool that can help you do that. When you go on any journey, you need appropriate tools along the way. Because of the very practical nature of certain aspects of nursing, you already have the most important tool you'll need. Think about it...change involves identification and assessment of the problem, planning, systematic action, and evaluation. Recognize these steps? It is the *nursing process*. Now is your chance to turn the nursing process *inward*. How wonderful to be able to use all of the information you had to memorize in nursing theory classes to create the kind of life you have always wanted!

Nurses use the nursing process in order to understand the complexities of each patient and to develop and implement effective plans of care (*changes*) for them. This same process can be used to help you understand your *own* complexities — your likes, dislikes, values, dreams, and goals — and to develop an effective plan of life change for *yourself*. When nurses assess a patient, they look at the presenting problem, take a history (physical and emotional/mental), and perform various assessment skills to gather information about the patient's condition. This information is then used in planning care that will facilitate recovery, independence, and a return to optimal health for the patient. All nurses learn to do this. But how can you use this nursing process on *yourself*?

The steps are really the same. First, the presenting problem must be identified. Most nurses would probably agree that change — or, more specifically, how nurses *react* to the rapid changes in health care — is the presenting problem. In this book, change issues are discussed in Section 1.

Once you identify the problem, the next step is to do an assessment and take *your own* history: physical, emotional, and mental. In Section 2 you'll learn to use your assessment skills on yourself to record your history and gather the information you need to develop a plan for finding optimal health and happiness in your work.

In Section 3 you'll begin to use your planning skills to look at your available options, set your goals, and develop a *plan for your future*.

But even the best-laid plans are worthless if they cannot be implemented. In Section 4 you'll learn the "rules of the game," and begin to see that your skills in carrying out, or implementing, a plan of action go far beyond the realm of patient care! They can be transferred to the realm of *self-care!*

If you make the commitment to yourself to work with the information and steps in this book, it will guide you through your own career development process. Each step builds on the last, and it is not always easy. I had tremendous resistance to working with this material. These exercises had been suggested to me, in various forms, for years before I became desperate enough to try them. It was like pulling teeth to get me to actually sit down and evaluate my career path, the choices I've made, and the degree of happiness I experienced each step of the way. I didn't think I could allow myself to daydream about my ideal career opportunity. But I surprised myself.

While going though the steps, the value in this seemingly mundane and time-consuming process became apparent. Soon, the direction I wanted to head became clearer. Then, after much weeping and wailing and gnashing of teeth, I got up the courage to do some informational interviewing. It was terrific! The picture was getting clearer and clearer. The goals were written down, and soon I had a plan! And if anybody knows how to work off of a plan, it's a nurse. I was off and running!

It may feel like a long and arduous process, but it is so much more than just getting a plan together. You are in the process of owning *you:* of valuing yourself enough to pursue your dreams; of increasing your sense of self, enlarging your world, and developing a feeling of personal empowerment; and of building the kind of career you always sensed you wanted but were never able to picture. Certainly a worthwhile endeavor!

Current Changes in Health Care

Problem or Opportunity?

CHAPTER 1

Health Care Reform

Have you ever felt like the nurse in this picture? Ever felt like "health care reform" was this huge, overpowering political force threatening to shatter your working world? The entire health care industry seems to be reeling from the rapid-fire changes that have occurred in the past five years. Many nurses are feeling confused by all the political rhetoric, frightened for their job security, and angry at a "system" that makes changes quickly and seemingly without recognizing the value of the central role that nursing plays in health care delivery. Many nurses say that keeping up with and participating in all the changes is just too much to deal with. They feel it is "out of their hands," and try not to think about it.

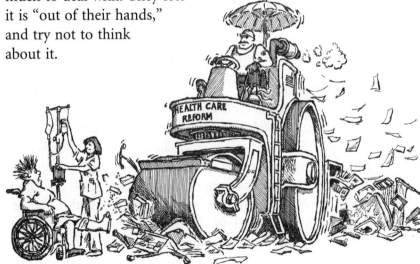

Health care in America is evolving into a new model that just doesn't fit into the same shell as the old one. This evolution is fueled by many different sources: breakthrough scientific discoveries and a cultural shift toward valuing health and wellness, as well as political agendas and corporate bottom lines, to name just a few. And, as with any great evolutionary shift, what initially feels like a shattering of the world as we know it brings in its wake tremendous possibility. Viewing health care reform from a broad, historical perspective helps to reveal this evolutionary potential.

Historically, nursing schools focused on bedside skills. You did your clinicals in the hospital and were sent out into the working world with a strong belief that the key to your success lay in providing hospital-based bedside care. This is, of course, the traditional "face" of nursing. And, quite possibly, hospital-based care is what you enjoy, what you *know* you do well, and what you *want* to do. There are many nurses who prefer this setting, who love the challenges and the patient contact, and who see the current changes as not so different from those that took place 5 or 10 or 20 years ago. Few workplaces offer the professional challenges, good income, benefits, and flexibility of scheduling that hospital nursing offers. In today's busy double-income-family world, these are not small issues for many people. The satisfaction of working with the acutely ill patient is exactly what millions of nurses want and enjoy.

The hospital has always been an arena for change. Just 40 years ago there was no such thing as an ICU, open heart surgery, or electronic blood pressure cuffs and thermometers. Even disposable needles did not exist! Rapid technological advances and shifts in patient care delivery models (such as the shift from team nursing to primary nursing in the 1980s and now the shift back to a team approach) are just *some* of the changes nurses have been dealing with for hundreds of years—maybe even since their very first days in the hospital setting. Health

8

care reform may simply be the most recent in a long line of changes nurses have faced.

Whether it's called team nursing, patient-focused care, or case management, most hospitals are now implementing managed care programs to cut costs and streamline patient care. A central feature of most of these programs is hiring unlicensed assistive personnel to work with the professional nurse. This practice can dramatically change the nurse's role from one that provides comprehensive care of each patient to one that supervises a team of caregivers, appropriately delegating activities while maintaining personal accountability for the quality and safety of care. Unlicensed assistive personnel with titles such as Patient Care Associates or Patient Care Technician (I was recently in a hospital where they were called Nurse Extenders!) are assigned to an RN, or an RN and LVN/LPN team, and are there to provide direct care to patients. Looking a lot like the team nursing of the 1970s and early 1980s, this is a BIG change from the primary nursing push of the mid-1980s and early 1990s, in which the all-RN staff provided comprehensive primary care to patients, sometimes with 24-hour accountability!

Appropriately utilized unlicensed assistive personnel, or UAPs, could eliminate the problem of nurses having to perform clinical duties beneath their skill levels—a great source of frustration for many nurses. Studies have shown that RNs are greatly underutilized. Research by the New Jersey Department of Health in the 1980s, the height of the primary nursing push, indicated that 23% to 48% of nurses' time was invested in work inappropriate to their role. Utilization of UAPs could allow nurses to apply more of their training to assessing, planning, implementing, and evaluating care of the patient. The role of the nurse as patient advocate, systems coordinator, and integrator of the total hospital experience is logical and cost-effective. There is great potential here for increased job satisfaction and professionalism for the nurse.

However, when UAPs are inappropriately utilized, problems are inevitable. A major risk is that not enough RNs would be present to provide high quality care. More than half of the state nurses' associations have reported instances in which staff mix ratios were unsafe. Many nurses in this situation perceive themselves not as professional case managers directing comprehensive care of the patient, but as IV-hanging pill-pushers without enough time to interact with their patients. This situation could seriously undermine the nurses ability to provide the skillful clinical management that has been associated with shorter hospital stays, less need for costly testing, and optimal coordination of hospital services—all of which are critical to the financial integrity of hospitals.

Nurses are often forced to deal with factors which affect their practice but are completely beyond their control. The industry is reacting to the shrinking health care dollar, government regulations, new medical technology (the use of which has tripled in the past decade!), shifts in patient population, alternative staffing patterns, and increased patient acuity. Rumors circulate about downsizing, reorganization, restructuring, work system redesign (or even "work transformation," as it was so nicely called in one hospital I recently visited)...need I go on? Clearly, survival in the hospital setting depends on the ability of each nurse to accept and adapt to change.

For all of the reasons discussed above, traditional roles and expectations for nurses continue to break down—breaking the mold, if you will, that cast the traditional nurse. The shift away from hospital-based health care delivery is well documented. While the *number* of nurses working in the hospital setting continues to grow steadily, the *percentage* of nurses working in the hospital setting has decreased from 67.9% in 1988 to 66.5% in 1992—a total of 1.4%, which is more than 17,000 nurses (Dept. of Health and Human Services, Division of Nursing). There was a 15% reduction in patient care beds in the nation's hospitals between 1980 and 1993 (U.S. Bureau of Census, 1995). Nurses have been downsized, outsourced, restructured, cross-trained, and even laid off as a result of the health care industry's scramble to provide more care to sicker patients while decreasing costs. Newly graduated nurses are often struggling to find their place in an industry that no longer guarantees a position in the hospital as their first job. Out of sheer necessity, you, as a nurse, are now faced with a myriad of choices as to where you can go to work.

While many nurses will continue to pursue work in the challenging hospital arena, or in the outpatient or home care setting, an increasing number of nurses today are working in health-related, non-traditional nursing environments. Some of these people do not consider their work nursing, while others clearly do. Nonetheless, as nurses increasingly enter fields such as insurance, law, sales, and consulting—or even become entrepreneurs, opening businesses of their own—they are re-creating nursing and recognizing its enormous potential. No matter what career choice you make as a nurse, you carry the philosophical threads of nursing into that career. Nurses in insurance or law carry the same fundamental body of knowledge into their work that med/surg or home care nurses carry into theirs. Within this simple fact lies great power to transform health care, medicine, law, insurance ... any arena in which you choose to work! Suddenly, the possibility exists for you to redefine yourself and nursing, to change the course of your future, to explore opportunities that did not exist before.

The problem is, how do you find your way through this new terrain to determine where you belong?

For years, I would get so frustrated when people would say things like, "There are so many opportunities out there for nurses. You should go into ..." I don't know about you, but my nursing program did *not* include a semester on health care reform, marketing, *or* career planning. I didn't have any idea how to find all those opportunities everyone was telling me about! Of course, these topics *are* covered in nursing programs today, but back then the need to include career development in the nursing curriculum was far less important. Issues such as reimbursement, reform, and reorganization did not have a direct impact upon nurses. But then along came DRGs, followed shortly after by talk of health care reform and the waves of change that are now being experienced full force — *big* changes that have bowled over more than a few of us. Well, maybe it's time for nurses to pick ourselves up, dust ourselves off, and figure out where we fit in this new model of health care!

In spite of how confusing these changes seem, and how unpredictable and out of control health care reform may feel, it is important to recognize this time as an opportunity for nursing to evolve and assume a new role in health care for the 21st century — a role that reflects the practical and philosophical foundations of nursing as an entity in itself, rather than one inexorably intertwined with the world of medicine. It is time for nurses to stand side by side with other health care professionals — including doctors — and make our contribution with pride!

It is said that power is the ability to influence change. If nurses step forward and assume leaderership roles in the health care industry of the 21st century, we can become vastly powerful change agents. This may sound like a daunting task. But the truth is that any evolutionary change takes place individual by individual, at least at first.

In her book, *On Specialization in Nursing: Toward a New Empowerment,* Margretta Styles, the ex-dean of the School of Nursing at the University of California in San Francisco, makes a distinction between "professionhood" and "professionalism."

She describes professionhood as the individual characteristics of any one member of the profession and professionalism as the composite character of the profession. She strongly believes that in order for nursing to achieve professionalism, profession-hood must precede it. As each nurse accepts responsibility for their own individual contribution to the profession, then the entire profession becomes empowered.

You can contribute to that evolution by becoming the person, and the professional, that you have always wanted to be. The trick is to know who you are, where you want to go, and how you can get there. Today's requirements for success include a careful examination of where your skills, personality, temperament, and drive could be best put to use—where you could find "a good match."

The day that each of us is able to stand tall and proud of our profession, reflecting ourselves in a positive light to others, will be the day that the full potential of nurses will finally register with other nurses and health care consumers alike. It is more important than ever that we make clear and positive choices in our work, find our niche in the many options that exist, and reflect our excitement and happiness with our profession out into the world. It is equally important that we treat ourselves and each other with a respect born of professionalism and a sense of esteem. In this way, members of the entire nursing community can begin to feel proud to associate with each other and can build on our already rich and diverse heritage.

CHAPTER 2

Change Management
Hang on for the ride of your life!

I was 31 years old when I went to Disneyland for the first time. My friend Ruth, who was raised in Southern California and had been to Disneyland hundreds of times, was shocked that I'd never been there and insisted that I'd *love* it. I was skeptical. My stomach lurched with the memory of a harrowing encounter on the Zipper at the county fair when I was just 15. It had been one of life's more embarrassing moments, as I heaved into the bushes with all my high school friends waiting nearby.

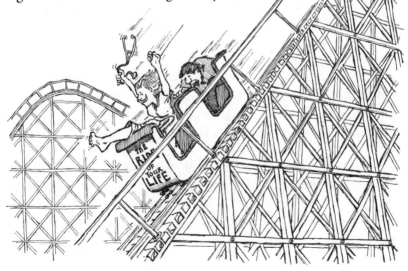

15

Certainly not interested in a repeat performance of *that* spectacle, I had never gone on another ride! Needless to say, going to Disneyland, with its huge roller coasters and all those spinning rides, had been out of the question. But Ruth's enthusiasm was contagious (and her insistence that I'd enjoy myself was relentless), so I decided it was time to try something different. With a scopolamine patch behind my left ear and my mind open to new adventure, I put myself into the capable hands of this self-appointed Official Disneyland Guide, and away we went.

I had the time of my life! The exhilaration of the rides was something I had never known before. The Matterhorn and Mr. Toad's Wild Ride were my personal favorites. As we rode them for the second time, it occurred to me that, because of one bad experience, I had deprived myself of all kinds of fun for more than 15 years! Never one to miss the opportunity to find profound meaning in each experience, it also occurred to me that life—and nursing—are a lot like the Matterhorn: a huge roller coaster ride with lots of unpredictable twists and turns. And like it or not, I was strapped into a seat and *not* in control of the ride. That left me a couple of choices: (1) hang on tight, ride the waves, and try to enjoy the exhilarating speed of the ride, or (2) hang on tight, fight the waves, and scan the nearby area for bushes.

But surely life (or nursing, or change) is not *really* like a roller coaster ride ... or is it? Since your reactions to change directly affect any choices you make in planning your career, it is in your best interest to understand the nature of change.

It is certainly not news that the nursing profession is undergoing radical and unpredictable change at this time. Change has become a fact of life for nurses—one that directly affects our day-to-day work in the world. Patient acuity has changed, methods of care delivery have changed, roles and responsibilities have changed. There is no way around it—change is here. The challenge is to understand that change *in and of itself* is not the problem. The Zipper was not the problem back in 1976 ... the way my stomach reacted was the problem! Change is simply a principle that is basic to the universe. It is a process that does not have an identifiable beginning or end; rather, it is a series, an evolution. As one change is being completed, another is beginning.

William Bridges, author of *Managing Transitions,* suggests that our focus be less on the change itself and more on the psychological process we go through as we put closure on the old and begin to embrace the new. He calls this the Neutral Zone—the "nowhere between two somewheres." (I think I spent a couple years in The Zone in the early 1990s!) It is the journey from one identity to another. Getting comfortable in the Neutral Zone may well be the challenge of the 21st century. Have you noticed that the changes seem to be coming faster and faster compared to a few years ago?

The way we react to change is based on our personal experience and individual circumstances, which form the foundation for our expectations, perceptions, and personal growth. For this reason, change may cause us to recall unresolved personal experiences from our past, which uproot anxiety and provoke family or work conflicts. It can be difficult to maintain a boundary between these past experiences and current situations.

It is important not to blame the changes—which are merely the trigger—for a lifetime of frustrations, but to keep proper perspective on which behaviors are a natural result of change and which are rooted in old, well-established patterns of behavior. This understanding is a key link to experiencing a healthy adaptation to change. It keeps us from repetitive, knee-jerk reactions that lock us into these old patterns and prevent us from making positive, growth-affirming change in our lives.

A person's style of managing change reflects their degree of self-confidence and sense of personal power, so you will see nurses managing change in a variety of ways. Some of us try to ignore the fact that it is happening. We dig in our heels and, determined to keep things the way they have been, resist the change and refuse to participate. Some may even try to sabotage the efforts of others. The problem with this method is that *there is no stopping change.* Just because you don't want things to change does not mean they won't. The change will happen all around you and, if you don't see it and deal with it, it'll most likely smack you in the head like a two-by-four every time you turn around. You may, someday, be *forced* to adapt to the change, and you will have had *zero* input into how it all came about. This is almost guaranteed to build anger and re-sentment on the part of the "forcee," and can make the work environment nearly intolerable.

Other nurses act as "intrapreneurs," or people who take hands-on responsibility for creating innovation within an orga-nization. They may seem to "roll with the punches," introduc-ing new ideas and adapting to change as if it were just a matter of course.

And there is an entire continuum in between.

In addition, the way in which the manager adapts to change frequently sets the tone for the entire staff and can have a pro-foundly positive—or profoundly *negative*—impact on how you and your peers deal with changes. All of these reactions to change come together to create a workplace that is varied and often unpredictable.

Even carefully planned and implemented change is dis-ruptive. It throws off our sense of "even-keel" functioning. Unplanned, frequent change does not give us time to adapt and increases our stress and sense of powerlessness over events that are affecting us. Reactions to change can take the form of uncertainty, anxiety, frustration, anger, rigid behavior, decreased objectivity, increased control over one's territory, possessiveness, and—probably the most frequent reaction— criticism of changes. Criticism may be one of the most insidious and powerful negative influences on people's ability to adapt to change. Have you ever had a workday turn bad because there was a nurse who kept criticizing and complaining about the changes that had taken place, continually reminding all the rest of the staff that they, too, may have preferred it the "old way"? Soon everyone is cranky, fed up, and complaining just as loudly. Although it is never *easy* to change behaviors that stem from an entire lifetime of experiences, your attitude is one aspect of change that you *can* control.

Reframing, or altering, your view of change can be a profoundly effective way of dealing with negative interpretations of disruptive change. In fact, possibly the greatest influence on how you deal with change is how you frame the event. For example, do you feel this is the best time ever to be involved in health care and see the changes as exhilarating and fun, like a roller coaster ride? Or do you feel as if the sky is falling and that nursing as a profession is going down with it? Each of these "frames of reference" sets the tone for your thoughts, feelings, and reactions any time you are confronted with new changes. Making a simple change in your frame of reference will have a profound impact on your thoughts, feelings, and reactions when you encounter change.

The value of reframing your views about change is that it helps you to find the power in adversity. Without change, perhaps we would never discover our potential, or be asked to step beyond our usual safety zone. Ask yourself: Is there any less destructive way to look at this change? Is there anything positive that could occur because of it? Re-focusing and re-framing the event can help you find the energy to take the next few steps as you make your way through the adjustment phase.

For example, maybe getting laid off—or even the *fear* of being laid off—could provide the incentive needed to start the career you'd always dreamed of having. I recently ran into a woman I worked with in the perinatal department of a local hospital. She had worked part-time in the nursery and part-time as the hospital educator. She told me that on the very same day she received word that she was to be laid off, she saw an ad in the newspaper for a position with the county providing health care and counseling for pregnant teens—just the type of work she'd always wanted! She loves her new job and is happy to have made the change.

Being laid off worked out well for this woman, as it does for many others. But change and layoffs do not always have a happy ending, and they do not tend to be a favorite topic of conversation for most people. The truth is, sometimes it is just plain hard to deal with change. In fact, at this point you may be tired of all this talk about change, change, change, and may feel depressed or angry—you may even be thinking about putting this *#! #**%! book down for good! Well, take heart, it's not all bad news!

Change is not something that merely happens. It is an activity in which you actively participate. It could be positive, it could be negative—but you *are* participating. Even digging your heels in is participating. Yes, change affects our lives every day. Often, it seems to make things more difficult. But, our *choices* determine the final outcome of any situation we face. Participating in the creative act of change and being an active force in our development involves risking to choose.

To choose is to give up the comfortable old for the uncertain new. To choose is to define and shape, to delineate and make clear. Our choices are what define us as individuals. We have the opportunity to make choices that can greatly improve our quality of life. Even those of us who feel trapped by life or work circumstances are making a choice, whether it's to improve our situation or "wait and see" what happens.

My wise friend Susan once said to me, "When you feel stuck, do just one thing differently." These words have come back to me over and over. Sometimes even the smallest inner change of direction or attitude can break things loose and open doorways you never thought would open for you. Maybe you basically like your job but have been unhappy recently. Choosing to make a small change or a series of small changes —like becoming a preceptor, helping design the new home-care patient intake forms, or taking some new classes—could be just what you need to realign yourself with your current job and rediscover what you *like* about your situation. Or perhaps you are ready for an entirely new career direction. Sometimes, simply the clear realization that you *want* to make the change works as a catalyst and propels you through the steps required to bring it to fruition.

Daryl Conner, author of *Managing at the Speed of Change,* says, "The secret to mastering greater levels of change is not to press harder on a pedal already floored, but to shift gears." Do one thing differently. Make some choices about what you can do to make the best out of a new (*or* old) situation.

One of the most effective ways of dealing with change is to become an *active* participant—a nurse *intrapreneur.* Being an intrapreneur is based more on a state of mind or attitude than personality characteristics. An intrapreneur is action-oriented, optimistic, self-determined, and willing to take initiative (Manion, 1991). A nurse intrapreneur might create innovation within the health care organization through the introduction of a new product, a different service, or simply a new way of doing something. Even something simple, such as keeping current on issues in health care, allows you to anticipate how you can influence and participate in upcoming changes. This knowledge can put you in a position of being able to *act* rather than *react*. I know, I know—you're probably saying, "But there's too much going on in my life already. I don't have the time, and besides, I don't *want* to participate. I just want to put in my eight hours and go home." This may be true. But the days of just "putting in your time" may be gone.

These days, nursing, like most professions, is requiring a different kind of commitment from its members. It requires more active participation: more input from staff on how to reduce the budget, implement new patient care models, deal with more and more unlicensed professionals, meet this month's sales quota, revise standard-of-care guidelines to meet new insurance reimbursement schedules. Remember the days when the word "budget" *never* came up in a conversation between nurses? Well, those days are gone. And without your input, what you are potentially left with are new plans that do not work in real life. Sounded good to the "suits," but doesn't work for the "scrubs." Ever seen that happen?

The good news is that participating more actively as a change agent gives you the opportunity to deal with your own and other people's reactions, claim your independence, and "own" your creativity—do things *your* way, with *your* flair. Also, the energy and excitement that result from seeing ideas for improved patient care, education, and other nursing services implemented and working is profound. The same parts of you that gain satisfaction from having an impact on the lives of your patients can feel a powerful sense of personal satisfaction from having a broader impact on the lives of many.

Even a few hours of participation a week can go a long way toward improving the implementation of change. Serve on some committees or volunteer to do some research on how other institutions have managed similar situations. A few phone calls may be all it takes to gather the information that can guide

22

your unit to making change work. Even just offering your feedback to your manager (I said *feedback*, not complaints) can make you feel as if you are participating in the change process. Objective information accompanied by suggestions goes a lot further than statements such as, "I can't stand this new charting method. It *stinks*, and I'm not going to do it." Instead of spending your lunch hour in a gripe session, spend some time discussing what is going on and brainstorming some workable solutions.

These are difficult tasks, I know. A common response to enforced change is the tendency to become demoralized, negative, and angry. It is never easy to keep a positive attitude in the face of disruptive change. But dealing with the current changes in nursing reminds me a lot of surfing (on what can seem like *tsunamis*, or large tidal waves): you will do much better riding the waves of change as they come than you will trying to stop them.

SECTION 2

Assessment

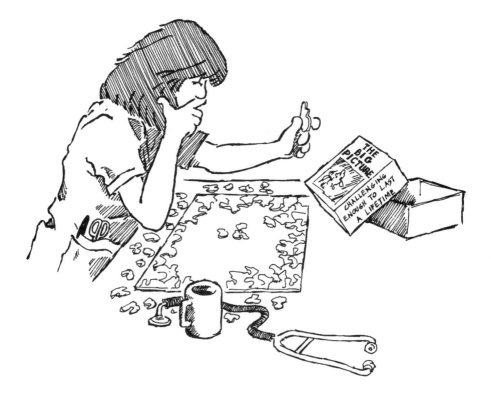

CHAPTER 3

Your Self-Assessment

Putting the pieces together

> *If you really know what things you want out of life,
> it's amazing how opportunities will come to enable
> you to carry them out.*
>
> – John M. Goddard

In Section 1, discussion centered around the *problem:* health care reform, change, and change management. It is important to have a clear understanding of these issues because the more clearly you can define the problem, the more easily you can tailor your plan of action to your specific needs. Having clearly identified the problem, you can now move on to the assessment phase and become clearer about your reactions to change, your history, values, ideals, and life priorities. This is a crucial step as you begin to identify what it is that you enjoy doing and what you most *want* to do with your future.

The following exercises are designed to get you thinking about what you have done in the past, what you most enjoyed doing, what your greatest achievements are, and what you want to do in the future. This information will then become the foundation upon which your goals and personal action plan are built. Gathering information on yourself and using it to put the pieces of *you* together is what enables you to find "the right match" and create the future you *really* want.

How many nurses do you know who work in an area of nursing that just isn't right for them? Years ago, there wasn't much thought given to *where* you were suited to work. Most of the time, if you were clinically competent, you could walk into a hospital and get hired. Where you went to work depended on where there were openings. Or maybe, like me, a childhood fantasy took you into an area of nursing that did not work for you in the long run.

As far back as I can remember, my dream was to be a nurse. Specifically, I wanted to be a critical care nurse. Every spare moment in nursing school was spent studying critical care. Nearly all of my clinical rotations were done in ICUs and ERs, and I enjoyed every minute of it. The technology and challenge appealed to me, as did what I perceived to be an aura of prestige around the critical care setting.

When I got my first job in ICU, it was as if I had landed in heaven. I loved it and worked hard at becoming an excellent critical care nurse. The crowning moment was the first time I made it all the way through a code blue without my hands shaking. What an achievement!

But, as the years went by, it became more and more difficult for me to be around such acutely ill patients and such extreme intervention. Thus began the long process of trying to reconnect with my feelings (and my shaking hands!) which I had numbed out in order to do my job.

Years after I finally left the ICU setting for good, it occurred to me that I never really gave any thought to examining what type of nursing *suited me:* my personality, goals, and dreams. I do love technology (I'm basically a techno-geek at heart), but I also love to connect with people, to acknowledge and honor their experience (even if that experience is suffering), and to do what I can to alleviate their pain and facilitate health and independence. This was a daunting task in the critical care setting, where suffering and pain are so much a part of each day, and health and independence often don't even enter the picture.

I'm not saying my choice was a wrong one. The years spent in the ICU were valuable contributions to my life and the lives of many others. But perhaps if I had paid attention, realized how transferable my skills were, and given careful contemplation to what other arenas interested me, I would have known better and not stayed beyond my tolerance point.

Working with the exercises in this chapter helped me to find a career that appeals to my love of technology and writing, allows me to connect with nurses from all over the country, and gives me the opportunity to guide the way through the change process. Not what I envisioned in nursing school, but a *good* match for me and what I most enjoy doing. Whether you end up choosing a staff nurse position on a med-surg floor or starting your own Burmese restaurant, the only way to be *sure* it is what you want is to *look carefully at what you want.* A key to that process is knowing what you have to offer. And *most* of the nurses I've spoken to in the past several years have no idea how valuable—and *transferable*—their skills and training are.

The U.S. Bureau of Labor Statistics publishes the *Occupational Outlook Handbook,* in which more than 200 occupations are organized by interest and job title. These occupations are then compared in terms of job requirements, work environment, and occupational characteristics. An examination of the job requirements, or "universal" job skills, listed in this publication sheds some light on exactly *how* transferable nurses' skills can be. The job requirements are:

1. Leadership/persuasion
2. Problem-solving/creativity
3. Working as part of a team
4. Manual dexterity
5. Helping/instructing others
6. Initiative
7. Frequent public contact
8. Physical stamina

Of more than 200 jobs, nursing was one of the *very* few professions that was identified as requiring qualities from *all* eight skill areas! (The other professions that required all eight qualities were teachers; physical, recreational, and occupational therapists; and police/EMTs. No big surprise here, right?) In addition, according to the U.S. Bureau of the Census, nursing jobs are predicted to increase 35 to 43% between 1992 and 2005.

Now, what may seem like only numbers and interesting bits of information actually speak *volumes* about skill transferability for nurses. So many times I've heard people comment that nurses can be put into almost any job and do it well. This is why: Nurses draw on skills that are very general to do very specific things. How many times have you gathered a key piece of information on your patient not from the chart, but from a "casual" conversation with a family member? How often have you found a creative solution to a seemingly insurmountable problem, such as teaching a woman crippled by rheumatoid arthritis to mix up and administer her own IV antibiotics by using any device that could be dreamed up to substitute for the painful lack of strength in her fingers?

Take a moment to look at each of the eight skill categories listed above. Think about how initiative, leadership, teaching, problem-solving, public contact, teamwork, manual dexterity, and physical stamina play a role in each and every moment of your work as a nurse. The perception that nurses can and do function well in a wide variety of settings begins to make sense. It also begins to make sense that nurses tend to be tremendous assets to the companies they work for by bringing a broad base of skills into every setting.

So now, with all of that in mind, it's time to begin the exercises! Don't be surprised if your "resistance alarms" go off. This may seem like a lot of work—and it is. But your work on these exercises will provide you with foundational information essential to making the right choices and planning change in your career. This information will be a guiding force as you move on to Chapter 4 and begin examining your career options. If you are only drawn to do some of the exercises, or if you feel very clear about what you want to do after completing only a few of them, feel free to move on to Chapter 4. But don't cheat yourself out of this process—it can be not only enlightening, but fun! You'll need a journal or notebook that you can use for the exercises involved in this process. For all the computer lovers in the crowd, put it on your computer—play with it and make it fun! Think of it as a game or a puzzle, and identify all the pieces that have made up the *you* in your professional path. Make an afternoon of it. Put on some tea or hot chocolate, or maybe your favorite tunes. Free yourself from distractions and *just DO it!* Getting started is the hardest part. Ready, set—GO!

EXERCISE 1: YOUR REACTIONS TO CHANGE

To be a successful change agent, you must understand how change affects you personally, what your areas of resistance are, and how you can deal with them. Examining your reactions to change is a vital first step in the process of developing and implementing a career plan. Take some time to reflect on the changes you have faced in the past few years and how you have reacted to them. Identify how your peers reacted and try to identify the agents of change in your workplace. You may want to use the format below as a guide. Try not to think of this as a chore or a test. It is the starting point for you to come to a better understanding of yourself and your reactions so that you can figure out how to make change into your ally. Have fun with it, and be totally honest!

First, identify what changes have occurred in your workplace in the past few years. In your personal life? Write them on a sheet of paper using the format below. This information can then be used to analyze your responses to change and how you view the advantages and disadvantages of these changes.

Changes I have gone through in the past few years	How did I react personally?	What were the advantages and disadvantages?

As you examine your responses to change, identify how your resistance to change manifests in your behavior.

▲ What, if anything, would you have done differently?

▲ What are some of the effective ways that you have dealt with change?

▲ What are some of the ineffective ways that you have dealt with change?

▲ Is there any one type of change (in the workplace or in your personal life) that is hardest for you to deal with?

Identify three areas you would like to work on to find more creative and self-affirming ways of adapting to change.

You may want to write them as if you were writing short-term/long-term goals for your patients. (For example: I will participate on at least one committee that is involved in planning the next change in our department.) These can be used later in Chapter 6, when you work on setting your short-term and long-term goals.

EXERCISE 2: VALUES CLARIFICATION

No proper discussion of career development can begin without first conducting a careful examination of our values, which determine what we really want out of life. Cringe. When I first heard about this phase of career development, I became a bit uneasy. Figuring out my personal values required self-examination (aargh!), and insight, and time, and thought ... and why in the world was *this* important, anyway? "Values" was such a nebulous term to me. These were not something I could simply list and move on to the next step. How in the world could I make a list of something that I didn't even understand? But I finally became convinced (*after* I had completed my values clarification) that understanding my motivations and values was a crucial step in the development of my goals, which was in turn a crucial step in career development.

So what is a value, anyway? Aside from being the source of your motivation, your values are your highest priorities in life. They are uniquely yours, and they provide a solid core from which you operate. No matter how much change you experience around you, your basic values operate like a sort of psychological glue, anchoring you during times of change.

When you feel as if you are smack dab in the middle of the whirling dervish of change that is hitting the health care industry, it can sometimes be difficult to know what is right and what is wrong, what you should do, and how you should do it. Most nurses have learned to function under a fairly well-established set of rules (or organizational values) and a given way of doing things. When in doubt, check the policy and procedure manual, right? If only life came with such a manual! As these rules change or become less predictable, it is valuable to consider what is important to you, what you believe in: your values. These values can be very simple, such as the importance of being compassionate, or doing your best no matter what.

When the structures you have become accustomed to as "definers" of your function are no longer in place, your own values become the core around which you refocus your efforts and make sense of the changes. Have you ever felt this happen? Perhaps a hospital reorganization leaves you with two nursing assistants on your team rather than two RNs. The way you divide your work, delegate, and care for your patients is no longer the same. It may be different than the way you have done things for your entire career! After a certain number of days of grouching, many nurses come to the conclusion that "all I can do is the best I can do," and they begin to adapt to the changes. This is an example of a person using a core value (doing your best no matter what) to adapt to a change that they cannot control. Other people, with different values, may say, "These working conditions are beyond my comfort level, and I'm choosing to leave this job for that reason." Or, "This change is actually for the best. Now I can focus more on the aspects of patient care that I really enjoy." They are using their own core values to adapt to the change.

Because there are such dramatic changes occurring in health care, taking the time to assess your own values is more important than ever. It will help you get to the other side of what seems like chaos. When you are in touch with your values, change can happen all around you, but it cannot shake your core. To begin the process of identifying your values, set aside some time during which you can be alone, quiet, and introspective. Begin to write down ideas in your notebook or journal as they come to you. You may want to use the following commonly stated priorities and suggested questions as a guide.

▲ Commonly stated priorities:

Physical health	Spirituality/religion
Education	Intellectual development
Mental health	Justice/truth
Family/friends	Community involvement
Financial security	Fulfilling career

▲ Evaluate the highest priorities in your life. What are the things that are most important to you?

▲ Make a list of the things that are most important to you. Try to list five to ten values, or even more.

▲ Now prioritize the values by placing them in order from most important to least important. If you have a feeling that the reality of your life is out of sync with your values/priorities, a good way to determine which values are most important is to gauge your level of discomfort as you think about each of them. Rank the value with which you are the *most* uncomfortable as the most important.

This is not about sadism. Really! Think about it. If there is an area in your life that is extremely important to you, but which has been ignored (because of lack of time, other obligations, etc.), then there is a gap between what you value most and what you *do* in your day-to-day life. We are often aware of —and uncomfortable about—these gaps. But they provide an excellent entry point, a place to develop goals to elicit change. Honesty is important here, because this is the foundational piece for developing your personal action plan.

▲ Get several sheets of paper. Write each of your values at the top of a separate page. Under each value, describe the behaviors that would be ideal within the framework of the value you want to perfect. Ask yourself: "If I were living that value perfectly, what would my behavior be like?" This clarification process will provide you with value statements, which are vital to your planning process and later goal development.

A value statement is a lot like a behavioral objective. It is a clear, concise statement of expected behaviors. For example, if my stated value is physical health, then my behaviors might include things that maintain good health: exercise, proper diet, and adequate rest and relaxation. My value statement could be: "I walk at least one half-hour four times each week." Write value statements for each of your prioritized values.

Once you've identified your values and written your value statements, you are ready to use them as you develop your goals and formulate a plan of action. Put them aside for now, and continue your self-assessment with the remaining exercises.

EXERCISE 3: WORK HISTORY

This exercise can provide important information about the choices you have made and how aligned with your dreams your work has been. Every job has its pluses and minuses, but how often do you sit down and think about what those pluses and minuses were and how they had an impact upon the way you feel about yourself and your work? Here is an opportunity for you to step back and take an objective look at your work experience. Perhaps then you can broaden your view and see how all the years of hard work fit into the "big picture" of your lifelong career. This exercise will also help you put your résumé together later.

In your notebook or journal, turn the page the long way so you can make several columns with headings like the ones listed below. Note that work experience can mean community and/ or volunteer activities in addition to past employment. *Any* past experience can help you a great deal as you identify your likes and dislikes.

Work experience and dates	Title or job description	What I enjoyed most	What I enjoyed least	My most significant achievement or contribution

Next, answer the following questions:

1. What was your favorite work experience? Why?

2. What was your least favorite work experience? Why?

3. What was your most significant contribution? Why?

4. What was your favorite activity on your most recent job?

5. What did you find challenging or stimulating about your most recent job?

6. Go through your work history and compile a list of the skills or the "action words" you used to describe what you most enjoyed and what you consider to be your greatest achievements. For example, maybe you most enjoyed "assessing complex patients with a wide variety of disease processes" or felt your greatest contribution was "initiating a new preceptor training program for newly hired nurses." Your action words would be "assessing" and "initiating." When your list is complete, set it aside for now and move on to exercise 4.

37

EXERCISE 4: FAVORITE ACTIVITIES

One of the most powerful ways to begin to identify which activities light your fire is to get a very clear idea of what you most enjoy doing. Our past jobs have all encompassed a great many skills. Nurses, more so than most professionals, are asked to do many different things (usually all at once!), and our expertise ranges from highly interpersonal to highly technical.

The following list contains words that describe the skills and activities that are performed by nurses as they go about their day. It is designed to help you identify the *skills* that come into play as you perform seemingly routine and perhaps mundane tasks. As you examine this list, focus not only on your professional life, but your personal life as well. Look at any roles you play: in the family, at work, in the community, at church, etc. Write down any skills or activities that you regularly perform. Think about what you did on your last shift, and mark the items on your list that apply.

This process may be stretched out over a couple of days. During your workday, you may find yourself trying to figure out which skills are involved in the various tasks you perform. If you think of skills and/or activities that are not on the list, add them! *Truth* is what we're after here—not what is expected and not what we've been told by others.

In your notebook or journal, write down the activities that you have found most *enjoyable, fulfilling,* and *rewarding.* You may want to assign your favorite activities a special mark.

▲ *Analyzing information*
　　Evaluating plans of care
　　Evaluating projects
　　Establishing standards
　　Noting relationship between ideas and things

▲ *Artistic*
  Creating things
  Designing things
  Eye for color/shape
  Interior design
  Landscaping

▲ *Assessing*
  Needs assessment
  Physical assessment
  Emotional assessment
  Group assessment

▲ *Being of service*
  Providing comfort
  Carrying out ideas
  Anticipating needs of others

▲ *Building a team*
  Working as member of team
  Delegating appropriately
  Assessing team values
  Working with needs and interests of others

▲ *Building/fixing*
  Working with tools/equipment
  Operating equipment
  Repairing equipment

▲ *Calculating*
  Working with numbers
  Record keeping
  Computing

▲ *Communicating*
    Listening to others
    Addressing groups
    Writing speeches
    Writing reports
    Interviewing

▲ *Coordinating*
    Doing several tasks at once
    Prioritizing
    Working well under stress

▲ *Evaluating*

▲ *Helping people*

▲ *Implementing a plan*
    Planning steps
    Establishing a timeline
    Delegating appropriately
    Evaluating progress, results

▲ *Inspecting*

▲ *Keeping records*
    Good at paperwork/filing
    Attention to detail
    Setting up systems

▲ *Leading*
    Showing initiative
    Recognizing needs of others
    Building a team
    Delegating appropriately
    Developing people
    Identifying problems

Solving problems
Making decisions
Motivating others
Building relationships

▲ *Managing others*
Supervising
Planning a project
Implementing change
Delegating/directing
Fostering staff growth

▲ *Observing*
Attention to detail
Able to see big picture

▲ *Organizing*
Data, people, events
Programs, materials

▲ *Performing (music, acting)*

▲ *Persuading/influencing others*
Selling ideas to others
Fundraising
Negotiating/bargaining

▲ *Planning*
Establishing objectives
Scheduling
Programming
Evaluating programs
Evaluating products
Developing policies and procedures
Preparing budgets
Developing goals/plans

▲ *Political/community work*
    Up on current events
    Aware of issues
    Knowledge of resources
    Public speaking
    Writing
    Community/political advocacy

▲ *Problem-solving*

▲ *Public speaking*
    Rapport with individuals and/or groups

▲ *Researching*
    Investigating
    Finding information
    Analyzing statistics
    Condensing information

▲ *Teaching*
    Explaining
    Preparing curriculum
    Precepting
    Acting as resource
    Public speaking

▲ *Working independently*

▲ *Writing*

Look closely at the items you've included on your list. Can you identify any patterns? Are most of the items you chose technical (researching, calculating, analyzing, keeping records, organizing, building/fixing, diagnosing) or are they based more in communication (helping people, creating, writing, teaching, persuading, communicating, being of service, public speaking, performing)? Do you notice a pattern of independence, an affinity for teamwork, or possibly a tilt towards management (planning, assessing, problem-solving, implementing change, leading, observing, speaking, team-building)? Do you perform the items you selected in your current job or are they totally different than what you are doing now?

Now, select your top five skills—those five activities that really make you feel alive, engaged, and happy when you are doing them. Rank these five in order of priority, with the one you most enjoy first. Give this all the time and thought you need—take yourself back in your mind to times when you were doing these things, and remember how you felt.

Put each of the five skills on the top of a separate sheet of paper. Now, write down at least two examples from your experience that describe your greatest achievement while performing these activities. What did you do? How did you do it? What was the result? This information will be helpful later, and you may find yourself referring to it when you are writing your résumé and cover letters.

EXERCISE 5: PERSONAL ACHIEVEMENTS

Make a list of your personal achievements. It has been said that a personal achievement is something that you did well, you enjoyed doing, and you are proud of. Think back throughout your lifetime, and remember the times when you did something that gave you a deep feeling of pride, satisfaction, and accomplishment. This can be associated with your work, family, school, community, childhood, social life—anything at all. It may seem insignificant to others, but what matters is how important it was to *you*. Don't be afraid to brag here.

Reach way back. Sometimes our greatest achievements occurred when we were very young! When I did this exercise, I was surprised to realize that achievements from my childhood and high school days were some of my most memorable and important experiences. It was also a surprise to see that the skills and activities that I enjoy most today are *directly related* to those early achievements. Entering adulthood can often mean a separation from childhood dreams and ideals, even though your foundations as an adult are laid by the experiences you had when you were a child!

Let yourself re-live the feelings of pride, joy, and accomplishment that you may have experienced in the achievements you identify.

For each achievement, identify the predominant activity or activities that were involved in your success. For example, if you were involved in successful contract negotiations at your hospital, you probably used skills like motivation and negotiation to succeed. If you were valedictorian for your class, you were most likely good at analyzing information, working independently, and studying (research).

As you look at your list of achievements, skills, and activities, examine it for *patterns*. Do your achievements have any similarities that may have spanned the years, recurring later and under different circumstances without you realizing it? Maybe the competitive side of you that won first place in the science fair during high school re-emerged years later when you won Nurse of the Year. Make note of any patterns or similarities you identify.

Now, correlate the list of skills and activities related to your achievements from above with the activities you identified as most enjoyable, fulfilling, and rewarding in exercises 3 and 4 by writing them side by side, in three columns labeled in the format shown on page 45. Arranging your information in this way allows you to examine what you really love to do, are proud of, and are good at from three different vantage points:

Exercise 3 Past work experiences	Exercise 4 Favorite skills and activities	Exercise 5 Greatest achievements

1. *Your past work experiences* (exercise 3), which identify where and how you have put your skills to work.

2. *Your favorite skills and activities* (exercise 4), which form the foundation for your greatest achievements.

3. *Your greatest achievements* (exercise 5), which are accomplished by utilizing your favorite skills and activities.

Backward and forward, forward and back. Although it may seem confusing at first, the goal here is to tap those parts of our memory that we can easily miss by using simple, intellectual exercises and list-making.

Are there any similarities or patterns that emerge? Are you utilizing the parts of yourself that you most value in your current job or in another part of your life, like the PTA or your church? How much of your day is spent doing things you really enjoy? Where are the gaps between what you *love to do* and what you *actually do*? Are there any ways to integrate the two so that you are doing what you love? Write down any thoughts or ideas you have during this exercise.

Take as much time as you need. You may find it valuable to go back over your data again at a later time. Maybe sleep on it, and look at your lists again with "fresh eyes" in the morning. The clearer you get about what you really love to do, the more likely you are to find a way to incorporate these activities into your daily life.

EXERCISE 6: WANT ADS

Go through the want ads in the Sunday paper, the *Wall Street Journal*, nursing magazines, job guides, online web sites, or other sources of employment advertisement you find, and carefully study what skills are required of applicants. Have a paper and pen ready, and begin to write down any aspects of these descriptions that you know you *can* and *want* to do. Do this for at least ten different ads. And *don't focus only on nursing jobs—read them all!* It doesn't matter if you qualify for the job or not. What you are doing is identifying skills and activities, and gathering ideas about types of work you could enjoy.

For example, it may be that while reading an ad for dean of a school of business (for which you are not likely to qualify), you identify activities that you *love* to do, such as curriculum development, teaching, budget development, or supervision. An ad for a writer/editor could remind you how much you enjoy writing reports, or creating brochures and newsletters. In this exercise, pull out only the tasks you love to do from many job descriptions, and see what job description you create based solely on what you love!

Scan your list and pick out your top ten skills. Rank them in order of priority (most favorite first). Compare this with the lists you compiled for exercises 3, 4, and 5. Do you notice any similarities?

Now, the *coup de grâce*. Combine the lists of activities from exercises 3, 4, 5 and 6. For example:

Exercise 3 *Past work experiences*	Exercise 4 *Favorite skills and activities*	Exercise 5 *Greatest achievements*	Exercise 6 *Want ads job description*

If you have any skills or activities that show up on more than one list, just cross them off so that you end up with one master list. From this list, select your top five favorite activities. Spend some time thinking about each of these activities; then rank them in order of priority. These top five activities represent a distillation of many years of hard work, of trial and error. They will provide a template for the goals you set later in this process by serving as a guide to ensure that your goals are in alignment with what you *truly* love to do. Write them on a separate page with the title "Master skills and activities list."

EXERCISE 7: IDEAL JOB/BUSINESS

Exploring your work history can give you a very good feel for where you've been, what you did "right" and enjoyed, and where you may have gone wrong in the past. It is equally valuable to stretch out into the future and imagine where you *could* go, where you would *like* to work, and form as clear an image of that as you can. These next few questions will ask you to speculate, to imagine, to dream—even to *make it up*! Don't underestimate the value of playing make-believe. Some of your best ideas may come out of a simple daydream!

1. Describe your ideal job. If you feel uncertain about what that would look like, pretend you are living in an ideal world, and make it up! Now is your chance to have it all! In which area or industry (not necessarily health care) would you most like to work? What area of the hospital, what type of product or service, what level of autonomy or teamwork would you prefer? Concentrate on all the details, such as duties, responsibilities, pay scale, work environment, geographic location, even what your co-workers might be like. Be sure to describe the contributions you wish to make and the results you want to achieve. The more detailed the better.

2. What, if anything, do you think could stop you from being able to have this job? Why?

3. If you identified a "stopper" in the above question, go back to your ideal world and describe what you would have to do to get past the obstacles, to clear the pathway for what you want in the workplace. Be specific.

4. If you could start your own business, what would it be? Remember, you are still in the ideal world, where anything can happen! Describe every detail of this business. Speculate on its growth potential and timeline for development. Where do you see it in one year? In five years? How do you see it fitting into its market? What population would it serve? What products or services would be involved? What would your role in the business be? If you find this a daunting task, just make it up! Now is your chance to put your dreams on paper!

5. What, if anything, do you think could stop you from being able to start this business? Why?

6. If you identified a "stopper" in the above question, go back to your ideal world and describe what you would have to do to get past these obstacles and clear the pathway for you to be able to develop the type of business you want. Be specific.

▲ ▲ ▲

Congratulations! Completing this section takes a lot of courage, introspection, and commitment. You can now refer back to these pages throughout the process of deciding your future direction. You may want to do the exercises again at some later date, if you feel that your priorities have changed significantly.

Use these pages as a resource when you feel off-track or when you realize you are spending all your time doing what you *have* to do rather than what you *want* to do. When it's time for your next New Year's resolution or a "tune-up" on your career plan or résumé, the information you just diligently recorded can be a real springboard for you, helping you to re-focus on what is most important to you.

You are now finished with the assessment phase and should be getting some idea of what you are looking for in a job. The next step is planning: examining your options, making choices, setting goals, and formulating a personal action plan to help you reach those goals. On to Section 3, which is devoted to the planning phase!

Planning

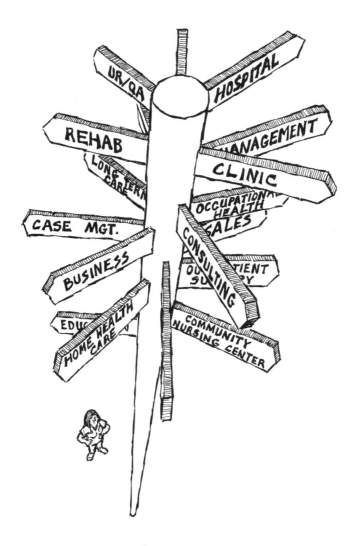

CHAPTER 4

Career Opportunities
Examining your options

In this chapter, a variety of career options will be examined. Believe it or not, there are *lots* of options for nurses, both in and out of the hospital setting. Now that you have given some thought to what you really enjoy doing, and what you are most suited to doing, scan through the following chapter and see if anything jumps out at you! Each of these options will be discussed in terms of job expectations, qualifications, advantages, disadvantages, salary, and/or general points of interest.

Keep your master list of skills and activities nearby (this is the list you compiled at the end of exercise 6 in Chapter 3). If any of the career options interest you, see if you can find a match between the skills required for that job and the skills you've listed as the ones you most enjoy using. You will find a comprehensive listing of resources appropriate to each option discussed in the resource guide at the end of this book.

Try not to bring any preconceived notions into this exploration. Many areas of nursing have had some kind of stigma associated with them or have been seen as "second best" to hospital care. Allow yourself to see these areas as if it's the first time you heard of them. No judgment, no commitment—just exploration.

INPATIENT CAREER OPTIONS FOR NURSES

▲ *Hospital-based nursing*

Many nurses still see hospital nursing as the epitome of clinical nursing. Although growth of hospital-based nursing is among the lowest in the industry at 5.5% (compared to home health, for example, which is growing at a rate of 38%), it still provides the working arena for 66.5% of the licensed RNs in this country. Fast-paced, clinically diverse, and challenging, this is an excellent arena for nurses who want to play a role in the care of acutely ill patients. Although there is a lot of room for lateral movement in this area (for example, from med/surg to ICU), and most hospitals have implemented clinical ladders for professional development, there is not much opportunity for upward advancement (for example, to management).

Many nurses choose to do a kind of "internal advancement" by becoming certified in their field of choice. For example, a nurse working in labor and delivery could become certified in perinatal nursing. The end result of this training and certification is a

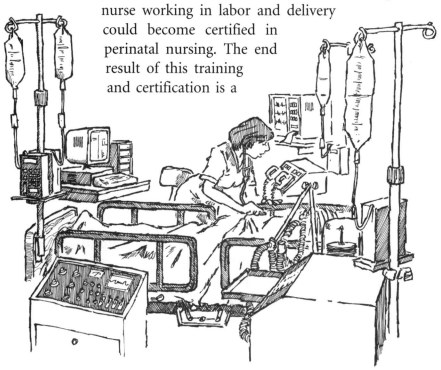

highly trained expert, who often advances up the clinical ladder, and serves as a resource, mentor, and/or coach for other staff members. Not only are certified nurses a tremendous addition to any unit, but they tend to have a higher degree of participation and satisfaction in the workplace.

Whether your interest lies in the highly technical role of the critical care nurse, the care of newborns in the nursery, or the fast-paced variety of the med/surg unit, one thing is certain: you will be experiencing change (and lots of it!) in your workplace. Change has become a fact of life in the hospital setting. There is a seemingly unending flow of new equipment and products; "better" flow sheets; progressive charting guidelines; and computer-based admission, discharge, ordering, monitoring, and charting. Hospitals are experiencing unprecedented severity of illness in their patients, accompanied by aggressive treatment both to speed discharge and to serve as appropriate therapeutic response to such acutely ill patients. Many of the basic patient care responsibilities are being performed by unlicensed assistive personnel. This means that more technical skills are required of registered nurses in literally *all* areas of the hospital.

Nurses who choose to work in the hospital setting (and more than 1.2 million nurses currently do!) are, by default, choosing to be front-line pioneers in a field of nursing that may currently feel more like a mine field than anything! Staff nurses walk with delicate balance between two seemingly conflicting priorities: quality patient care and cost containment. Both of these priorities are monumental in their importance and cannot (*will* not) go ignored. How do staff nurses "walk the line"? How can they navigate this terrain with integrity, using their skills and knowledge in the very best way possible? What impact will managed care have on the future of staff nursing and the delivery of quality patient care? The answers to these questions will be determined by the nurses who work in the hospital setting, more so than probably any administrative or governmental committee.

Staff nurses play an enormous role in determining the future of patient care delivery during perhaps the most exciting time in the history of health care. Over 1.2 million strong, these nurses are not to be ignored in the process of health care reform. Consider for a moment the impact 1.2 million nurses who have agreed to step forward, speak the truth, take risks, and *choose* to participate in the creation of their own future, could have on the process of restructuring hospital-based health care delivery in America! The possibility for nurses to become empowered professionals and play a profound role in ensuring quality patient care is very real.

Salaries for hospital-based nursing vary widely depending on your geographic location. The East and West Coasts tend to have higher salaries compared to the rest of the country. But no matter where you live, salaries tend to be good since the nursing shortage of the mid-1980s forced them higher. In fact, even though the 1990s have brought some decreases in wages and benefits, in-hospital nursing is still one of the best paid fields in which nurses can work at this time. The average salary for a staff nurse is $36,618, but you can expect the salary to range from $22,000 to $50,960, depending upon geographic location, years of employment, shift differentials, etc. (U.S. Department of Labor's Bureau of Labor Statistics, 1994).

▲ Nurse managers

Although management is still a viable career option in some hospitals, this area of nursing has undergone extensive change in recent years. Nearly all of the hospitals I've encountered in the past few years have experienced some form of downsizing, in which management positions were eliminated or consolidated. Managers have been asked to step down, "bid" for other positions within the facility, or assume broader management responsibilities, such as the addition of ancillary departments (for example, housekeeping or patient transportation) to their existing units. Advanced degrees are often required of the new manager, who serves a broader role within the hospital. While this was once the only upward advancement available for nurses, it has become less available with this new educational requirement.

For those nurses who are interested in management or business and willing to consider returning to school, this is a very exciting option. Complex budgetary guidelines, accreditation requirements, legal issues, and staffing changes provide the analytical, strategic thinker with many ongoing challenges! You can expect a salary range of $36,500 to $47,000, with an average of $42,589 (Department of Health and Human Services, Division of Nursing).

▲ Education and training

This area of nursing, like most, has shifted considerably over the past five years. There was a time when hospitals seemed to be drastically paring down or even eliminating in-house nursing education departments, often contracting with consultants to provide required education services. Nursing education was seen as an extraneous department that could be eliminated to save the cost of supporting a full-time staff.

But the most recent financial crunch affecting health care has forced a re-examination of the high cost of consultants, and nursing education has once again been taken in-house in many hospitals. Consistent education for licensed and unlicensed staff, safety instruction, and monitoring staff skill levels with regard to equipment have all become increasingly important to the hospital, and often the nurse educator is the one to oversee these functions.

Although this is not an area that employs a great number of nurses, if you have an interest in education you may be able to work yourself into a position by becoming an instructor in cardio-pulmonary resuscitation (CPR), advanced cardiac life support (ACLS), pediatric advanced life support (PALS), or neonatal advanced life support (NALS), and offering courses through the hospital. (Offering these courses is also a great way to become involved in community education.) Get involved by offering your input to the education department about up-coming classes, events, or projects. Offer to organize a seminar featuring an outside speaker or to assist in seminars sponsored by the hospital. Salary is comparable or slightly higher than that of a staff nurse.

▲ Utilization review / discharge planning / case management

Many hospitals and insurance companies now utilize nurses to do such things as pre-admission reviews, discharge planning, case management, and hospital stay review. Managed care or-ganizations and insurance companies may employ nurses as intake coordinators or case managers. These positions keep nurses involved in patient care, but in an entirely new way: as patient care advocates. You may be asked to review files and make recommendations regarding medical treatment, contact claimants, employers, and medical providers to clarify treatment and goals, and/or research and obtain cost-effective services and equipment.

This type of work requires a strong clinical background and good research and analysis skills. In this setting, nurses provide a bridge for patients and doctors between the clinical, or treatment, aspect of care and the business or insurance in-dustry. They frequently serve as a liaison between these two different worlds, helping to ensure that patients get the care they need and that no health care dollars are wasted on unnec-essary or ineffective treatments. Salary for this type of work is usually comparable to staff nursing, but may be slightly lower, depending on the setting.

▲ Risk management

This is usually a small department in most hospitals. Staff are responsible for tracking unusual incident reports, identifying potential areas of liability, educating staff on appropriate charting and reporting of incidents, and assisting in the event of any legal actions or malpractice suits. Working closely with quality assurance staff and possibly the hospital attorney, these nurses are responsible for investigating any incident that *could* end up in litigation, ensuring that all data is collected and coherent, and following up in the event of investigation, deposition, and/or lawsuit. It is a position that requires good organizational skills, persistence in enforcing policies, and the ability to present one's self appropriately with potential litigants and attorneys.

This area does not usually employ a large number of people. If you are interested in it, try talking to various risk management nurses to discover how you might break into the field. You may also want to contact the American Society for Healthcare Risk Management—they are listed in the resource guide at the end of the book.

OUTPATIENT CAREER OPTIONS FOR NURSES

▲ Home care

Described by the media as "the most rapidly growing sector in health care," home care has been receiving a lot of attention in recent years. The number of nurses employed in home care grew by 38% between 1988 and 1992 (Department of Health and Human Services, Division of Nursing). Reports indicate that national expenditures for home health care increased from $4.9 billion in 1985 to $20.8 billion by 1993. Medicare's spending on home care rose from less than $2 billion to more than

$10 billion in roughly the same period (Kellcher, 1996). The tremendous growth is rooted in a number of causes: technological advances allow more care to be delivered in the home, hospital stays are being shortened to meet fiscal constraints, and the number of elderly patients is steadily climbing. Most important of all, though: consumers often *prefer* home care.

Whether a large national chain, an agency affiliated with a hospital, or an independently owned and operated agency, there are thousands of home care agencies that serve in all areas of the country. The scope of these home care operations ranges from traditional, full-service agencies to organizations that specialize in hospice care, IV therapy, pediatrics, or fetal monitoring. This means there are opportunities for all types of nurses, from med/surg to pediatrics; perinatal to ICU. Home care is a great way for nurses to plan and provide direct patient care, but in a much more relaxed and autonomous setting than the hospital.

These nurses function as case managers, who see their caseload of patients as often as necessary. They may be asked to supervise unlicensed personnel, such as a home health aid, to ensure that the patient's needs for unskilled care are met. Psychosocial and family issues often need to be addressed and managed as a part of patient care. There is generally a great deal of patient/family teaching as the patient and family gradually assume responsibility for aspects of their care. Nurses in home care are often able to develop satisfying long-term relationships with patients and their families and can become a very important person in their lives. The atmosphere is casual, with most nurses wearing street clothes and delivering care in the patient's home rather than a sterile environment. Many nurses enjoy being able to focus fully on the patient without the constant distractions and interruptions that are usually a part of hospital nursing. It can be interesting and rewarding to witness the patients' growth in independence and empowerment as they learn to cope with their illness.

Generally a Monday-through-Friday position with little or no shift work and lots of flexibility and autonomy in scheduling your visits, this type of work appeals to many nurses who have families or a penchant for independence! Nurses check in at the agency at least once a day, with the bulk of the time spent in the field seeing patients. You may be asked to take turns carrying an on-call pager on weekends and nights. One drawback is the phenomenal amount of paperwork required, so if you dislike filling out forms or working on computers, beware!

Often a BSN and/or a public health nursing certificate are required to work in this setting. Pay does not tend to be as high as it is for hospital nurses, but many home health nurses say that the hours, working conditions, and flexibility are worth a slightly lower salary. According to the U.S. Department of Health and Human Services Division of Nursing, the national average is $32,621 annually.

Respect for cultural diversity is a must, since this type of nursing often requires visits to families of various ethnic backgrounds, and cultural practices can be strikingly different than those to which you are accustomed. Also, visits may take you into neighborhoods where safety is a consideration.

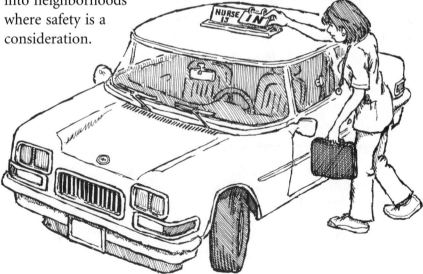

You might consider taking one of the many personal self-defense courses that are available. Check with your local police department or women's crisis hotline for recommendations.

▲ Long-term care

Although health care for the elderly spans a continuum from the hospital to a long-term care institution to home, the nursing home has come to symbolize long-term care for older people. Having endured the unfortunate stigma of being "second-class hospitals" and faced some very real problems with sub-optimal conditions, long-term care facilities (also called nursing homes or skilled nursing facilities) have not been considered an attractive career option for most nurses.

However, as the demographics of this country change, this area of nursing is changing right along with them. We are now confronted with a population that is older and more character-ized by chronic disease and disability. According to the Ameri-can Association of Retired Persons (AARP), more than 30 mil-lion people, or approximately 12.6% of Americans, are 65 years of age or older. By 2040 about 20% of the population will be 65 or older; 13 million of these will be over the age of 85. These shifts are the result of an increased life expectancy due to the successful containment of infectious disease and advances in the treatment of acute illness.

As the baby boomers are faced with providing health care for their parents, there is a sharp increase in attention focused on the types of care options that are available. The past trend of the elderly being cared for in the home, usually by a younger female family member, is no longer reality for most families that require two incomes. Higher quality health care for the elderly is being demanded by increasingly informed consumers.

Changes in federal law have forced radical improvement in the quality of care provided in long-term care facilities. The law requires these facilities to hire more registered and licensed staff and requires nursing assistants to be formally trained, to be certified by the state, and to complete annual continuing education courses. An Ombudsman program protects the rights of long-term residents and investigates any reports of misconduct. All of these factors have come together to greatly improve the conditions of long-term care facilities for patients and staff.

There are many advantages to working in this type of setting, not the least of which is that it is much less pressured and chaotic than the acute care environment. Patients are usually sent out of the facility if acute conditions arise. Death is often viewed as a natural life process here, without traumatic intervention to prolong the life of an elderly, chronically ill person. Long-term relationships are often developed between the nurse and the patients and their families, and the satisfaction of increasing the day-to-day comfort for the frail older person can be very rewarding. Usually the nurse supervises the LPN/LVN and certified nursing assistant (CNA) staff and is responsible for IVs, medications, treatments, and documentation. Working with a largely non-professional staff provides opportunities for mentoring, teaching, and team-building that can improve your professional esteem.

More and more facilities are managing younger patients, some with IVs, ventilator dependency, and tube feedings, as the insurance industry seeks new, less expensive ways to manage chronic patients. Facilities are increasingly being called on to provide services for a growing number of persons with AIDS and other terminal illnesses, a range of psychosocial and behavioral problems, head injuries, and people who need a period of convalescence or intensive rehab before returning home. As patient acuity rises, there is more and more clinical challenge for a technically minded nurse considering this area.

Because conditions in long-term care facilities vary greatly, it is extremely important to select a facility with values and professionalism that coincide with your own, at which you see opportunity for professional growth and development. Salary has traditionally been significantly lower than the hospital setting but is steadily increasing as demand for quality nurses increases in this area. According to the Buck Survey conducted by the American Health Care Association, the range is from $27,200 to $33,400 per year. The U.S. Department of Health and Human Services Division of Nursing lists the average income for nurses working in long-term care at $31,298.

This is a great career option for nurses who enjoy working with an elderly population and who want to participate in an area of health care currently undergoing tremendous reform. But then, aren't they all?

▲ Cardiac rehabilitation

Cardiac rehabilitation programs have been springing up over the past decade as the successful treatment of coronary heart disease has created a population of people in need of education and support in making lifestyle changes that help to prevent the worsening of heart disease. Usually located in a hospital setting, doctor's office, or fitness center, these programs utilize the expertise of registered nurses and exercise physiologists to provide a physical workout for cardiac patients while they are closely monitored to prevent overexertion and/or injury. The patient population includes post-op coronary bypass, valve replacement, heart cath, angioplasty, stents, and post-MI patients.

The nurse (most often with a critical care background) observes cardiac monitors during the exercise period and periodically checks pulse, blood pressure, and signs of exertion. There is usually an opportunity to teach relaxation and stress reduction. (It can be very exciting to guide a room full of 60-year-old Type A's through a meditation practice and witness their delight at such a foreign concept as relaxation!) Nutrition and lifestyle education and counseling can also be part of this job.

While this is not an area of nursing that employs great *numbers* of people, if you have an interest in cardiac rehab, try talking to local cardiologists to determine where existing programs are run or if there is enough need and interest to develop a new program. For critical care nurses, this can be a fun, part-time diversion that offers a chance to interact with patients who are on the road to recovery rather than in acute crisis.

▲ Rehabilitation nursing

Rehab nursing is rapidly developing into an extremely viable and attractive career option for nurses. Advances in the treatment of traumatic injuries have increased the number of patients requiring rehabilitation services; the number of facilities that provide services has *doubled* in the past decade (Hammers, 1993).

Chemical dependency and drug rehab programs employ a great number of nurses. While insurance companies are reducing payment for acute care, they are *increasing* reimbursement for the overall less costly rehab services. A recent survey showed that "every dollar spent on rehabilitation saves at least $10 on medical costs" (Hammers, 1993). With a wide range of patients, including people with chemical dependency, head injury, stroke, cardiac or respiratory conditions, amputees, and cancer survivors, there is a lot of variety and challenge for nurses who choose this area. Rehab units can be located in a rehab center, hospital, nursing home, or even the patient's home or work setting.

The focus of rehab nursing is to participate on an interdisciplinary team that works to help patients achieve their highest potential, adapt to their injury or illness, and increase their independence. Rehab nurses need to be excellent communicators, educators, planners, and team players. They will generally supervise unlicensed personnel and work closely with allied professionals in physical therapy, occupational therapy, and/or speech therapy to plan care for the patient and facilitate follow-through on new skills as they are learned. Nurses in this setting often become very involved in the lives of their patients and families, and can derive great satisfaction from participating in their patients' increasing independence and growth.

Training for rehab nurses is usually offered on the job. Some terrific resources are available through the Association of Rehab Nurses (ARN), which offers courses, books, audio and video tapes, and a program through which the nurse can become a certified rehabilitation registered nurse (CRRN). Salary varies widely depending on geographic location and the setting of the rehab center.

▲ Outpatient clinics

Nurses who choose to work in outpatient clinics often enjoy a more relaxed environment, providing care to patients with less acute conditions than those who are hospitalized. It usually means daytime hours and an entirely different view of patient care. Patients coming to a clinic could be there for preventative care, or they could be very sick. There are a wide variety of clinics available, ranging from standard medical and obstetrics clinics to holistic clinics and 24-hour acute care clinics. This variety allows nurses to choose an area that is in alignment with their interests. Often, clinic nurses work with only a few other people, and close friendships develop between clinic staff and physicians.

The pay for clinic nursing is usually significantly lower than hospital pay, but, as with the home care setting, many people are willing to accept a lower salary in order to enjoy the benefits of this setting. According to the U.S. Department of Health and Human Services Division of Nursing, the average salary for the ambulatory care setting is $27,949.

▲ *Outpatient surgical centers*

The number of outpatient surgical centers, or "surgi-centers," is growing rapidly as patients who do not require a post-operative hospital stay are being cared for in the far less expensive outpatient setting. Good nursing skills and resourcefulness are required in these jobs, as you do not have the "comfort" of having all the resources that are available in the hospital. This setting usually prefers to hire nurses who can scrub and/or circulate in the operating room as well as provide pre- and post-operative care. Consequently, this is a good option for people with experience in the OR; but don't count yourself out if you have critical care, ER, or even labor and delivery experience.

For many years, ORs—both inpatient and outpatient—have been difficult settings for new staff to break into. They have tended to be staffed by long-term employees, so training hasn't been offered for new employees. However, over 13% of licensed registered nurses are between ages 55 and 65 (Department of Health and Human Services, Division of Nursing), so as OR nurses now begin to retire and the outpatient surgi-centers continue to grow, training programs are once again starting to be offered.

As with most outpatient settings, you can expect the salary to be slightly lower than the hospital setting.

▲ *Community education*

There is a growing need for nurses to provide wellness education in various areas; subjects include prenatal education, weight management, smoking cessation, basic life support/ CPR, "Better Breathers" groups, and sex education. Talk to your Chamber of Commerce, local businesses, and community groups to see what programs are offered and where there may be a need for new programs. Contact the organizations listed in the resource guide at the end of this book to find out what types of programs they offer, how you might participate, or where they have identified a need in most communities. You may be affiliated with a doctor's office or health club, sponsored by a local corporation or store, or totally independent with your own place of business. There is a need to become established and respected in the community, to build a following and a reputation for providing quality education. Evening hours will probably be required to accommodate working participants, but you have a great deal of independence in setting your schedule. This could be an excellent opportunity to develop and grow your own business, as well as create a variety of different classes.

Other areas in the community that provide an arena for nurses interested in providing wellness education are:

- Mobile health screening (may be hospital-based, or in a mobile unit co-sponsored by a local department store, TV, or radio station)
- Homeless housing
- Rape crisis centers
- Sexual assault resource teams
- Recovery centers
- Planned Parenthood
- Children's programs

▲ Community nursing centers / community nursing organizations

One new trend in health care is the community nursing center, where care is provided to middle-class and/or poor patients at a cost lower than the standard outpatient setting. The possibilities for programs and services in this setting are vast. Nurses in this field are trained and skilled in many different modalities, including health education, patient teaching, stress control, weight management, nutritional education, parenting and childbearing education—the list goes on and on. There are now about 250 community nursing centers in the U.S. Refer to the resource guide for organizations to contact that may be of help in determining what services you could offer to your community.

An article by Thelma Schorr entitled "Nurse-Run Managed Care?" (written for the *American Journal of Nursing*) describes a project set up in the early 1980s by Phyllis Ethridge, vice-president for nursing at Carondelet St. Mary's Hospital in Tucson, Arizona. Ethridge established a managed care system that utilized "a professional nursing network with nurse case managers at the hub." Patients were referred to this network of nurses from a variety of sources, ranging from hospital-based nurses to physicians. Nurses functioned as the primary health care providers for these patients, arranging for whatever treatment was needed. When patients required a service that couldn't be provided by the network, they were referred to an appropriate provider, and payment was automatically authorized.

The immediate access to patients gave the nurses the opportunity to initiate proper treatment immediately, before the need intensified, and drastically reduced the cost of treatment. This kept patients from being admitted—and re-admitted—to the hospital. Patients were educated in the early signs of the symptoms of disease and potential problems. This resulted in a dramatic 60% decrease in the number of patient days in the hospital. This nursing clinic won a bid in 1990 to manage the care of 10,000 elderly patients in a "senior plan" of an HMO called Family Health Plan. Carondelet St. Mary's soon had four different contracts, and in January of 1994, they began a demonstration project that was awarded to them by Health Care Financing Administration—which put them in direct competition with HMOs!

The implications of these types of projects are immense, and they reflect the earliest stages of nurses moving into their natural place within the health care system. Developing a community nursing organization is, no doubt, a huge undertaking —and not for everyone. But what an exciting arena for the visionary mavericks out there!

▲ *Forensic nursing and sexual assault nurse examiners*

This is a fast-paced, clinically and emotionally challenging area of nursing which is (unfortunately) growing quickly. Forensic nurses work with victims of crime. They attend to the victim's injuries; identify, document, and photograph injuries and wound patterns; collect samples of hair, tissue, and body fluids; and put together evidence that may be used later in court. They often act as expert witnesses, explaining evidence and presenting what they found in their examination and treatment of the victim. These nurses often work on call and come into the ER when a violent crime survivor presents for treatment.

Having a nurse who is specially trained to deal with the physical and emotional consequences of violent crimes, such as domestic violence, child and elder abuse, and sexual assault, can be of great comfort to a person who has just endured a violent attack. It prevents the patient from having to deal with the chaos and numerous caregivers that are the norm in busy ERs. If this is an area of interest for you, contact your local police or sheriff's department to gather information on how they manage violent crime victims who are in need of medical treatment.

An excellent resource for nurses interested in forensic nursing is Sandra Goldstein, RN, MSN, of Forensic Nursing Services in Santa Cruz, California. She is a partner in this nurse-owned and -managed consulting and education company that provides services related to the issues of sexual assault and domestic violence and helps communities set up programs to deal with these issues. She can be reached at 408-427-9935 (phone/fax), or by E-mail at sleuthrn@aol.com.

NON-PATIENT CARE AND BUSINESS CAREER OPTIONS FOR NURSES

▲ *Quality assurance / utilization review / case management*

This is an area of nursing that was developed and has grown as a direct result of the impact of managed care and Medicare on the health care system. It is an expansion of the nursing process in which nurses combine skills in assessment, planning, implementation, and evaluation to determine the right level of care for the patient. They are evaluating care rather than giving it; performing a sort of "gatekeeper" function. Rather than working for only the hospital, you might work for an insurance company, a managed care company (such as an HMO or PPO), or a consulting firm that provides contractual agreements with any of the above.

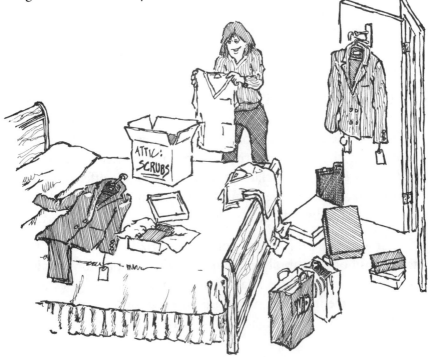

As an industry, this area has enormous growth potential as more stringent guidelines are established by managed care, Medicare, and even hospitals. Your duties would include reviewing medical records and activities, evaluating the need and appropriate level of care, and assessing the services provided, as well as the quality and timeliness of care.

This type of work requires a strong clinical background, an analytical mind, and the ability to perform research. It's often a desk job, where information is telephoned in to you. Occasionally you may be asked to meet with families or visit hospitals. You will get good business exposure with this type of work, and an overall picture of the issues involved in patient care. This kind of work tends to raise your consciousness about health care issues in general, increase your evaluative skills, and make you into a more well-rounded health care provider.

Disadvantages include a multitude of ethical dilemmas, such as working with complicated clinical issues and deciding who gets health care. It is a complex work arena with lots of liability for making wrong decisions. Often nurses miss the personal connection of the clinical setting and the "strokes" they used to receive from their patients.

Entry into this field is *definitely* made easier by obtaining appropriate education and training. Plus, it takes a lot of clinical skills to make the right choices and referrals. One of the main sources for the above information is Lonnie Friedman, owner of Quality Review Associates in Los Angeles. She offers a home study course for people interested in working in this field. It can be ordered by calling 800-562-2160.

Although there is large geographic variation, the salary for these positions is rapidly catching up with the pay for hospital nursing. One company I talked with in the Los Angeles area quoted their entry level pay at the low $40,000's, with potential to work up to the high $60,000's as a manager.

▲ *Occupational health and workers' compensation*

There are lots of different arenas in which to work in the field of occupational health and workers' comp. For example, in occupational health clinics nurses work at injury management, toxicology screening for environmental/occupational hazards (such as asbestos), providing educational services, and marketing their program to other industries. Their main source of contact is the employer, usually in employee relations. Workers' comp nurses, on the other hand, may be hired by: insurance companies, to perform case management for workers' comp cases; managed care groups, to provide case management services for PPOs and HMOs; or private companies, to manage the actual writing of policies for insurance agencies and keep financial losses down.

For example, Gari H. works in management for a workers' comp insurance company based in Minneapolis. She has seen the company's staff grow from 6 to 150 over the past nine years. They are opening new offices around the country to work with post-injury management. She reports that approximately 6% of the people involved in workers' comp claims cost 85% of the dollars spent. By identifying these high-risk injured workers and working closely with the employer to manage their recovery, her company provides an important service to employers, and also to workers who may never have had the type of support and guidance they needed to get back to work. Getting the employee back to work is a high priority, so workers' comp nurses work closely with employers to set up light duty work, which can break the cycle for people who, for a variety of reasons, *want* to be off work.

Some states have qualified rehabilitation consultants (QRCs) who are certified by the state and often hired by insurance companies to medically manage injured workers, help people find appropriate jobs after an injury, and work with long-term disability.

There is also an industrial nursing side to the occupational health arena. Nurses often provide teaching and training for corporations, such as airlines, in the areas of safety, basic CPR, and health maintenance.

There are a variety of ways to gain entry into these fields. QRCs are usually BSNs who decided to go to training courses and get certified, which provides an entry point into the field. Occupational health clinics may hire into an entry-level position, which creates the possibility of moving up in the ranks. Probably the most likely area for hiring nurses from the hospital setting is managed care—HMOs and PPOs. Gaining some experience in this setting can provide you with a springboard into the more competitive private companies. QA and UR experience is always a plus, so you may choose to start in these areas and move into the occupational health/workers' comp world.

Pay for this type of work is now competitive with pay in the hospital setting. It requires nurses who like to work on a team, have strong leadership qualities, good communication skills, and a sense of humor. Also important are a strong character, assertiveness, and professional demeanor, since most positions require you to do some sales to enroll new companies. Nurses must show initiative and have good problem-solving skills. It is a great area for people with a "maverick" mentality who are willing to take risks.

▲ Telephone triage and advice lines

Telephone triage is seen in a variety of settings including doctor's offices, HMOs, managed care companies, hospitals, clinics, and organized call centers devoted to health information and education. Nurses speak on the phone to patients, clients, or consumers, assisting them in determining the urgency of care needed, referring to or scheduling appointments with doctors, and providing health information and advice to callers.

These services are often started as marketing programs and are designed to provide general health information services to a community while making callers aware of services provided by local hospitals and physicians.

Triage services are an effective response to the rapid changes in health care. They provide services such as the management of demand for health services, recertification systems for insurance companies, support for managed care services, health information for consumers, education or counseling to a selected population, and after-hours programs for physicians. In addition, nurse consultation programs provide ongoing communication with high-risk populations in the home, such as those patients with chronic conditions and debilitating illnesses.

More and more insurance companies are offering this service to subscribers. It can save on unnecessary visits to the clinic and even the ER. Often, all people need is information—and nurses are perfect to provide this information in a clear way that patients can understand, since they are accustomed to providing patient education. Nurses in this setting use a computer program and enter the patient's complaint; then potential problems, explanations, and treatments show up on the screen. Believe it or not, there is an opportunity to develop relationships with some of the clients, since they may be frequent callers or you may set up a time for them to call back for follow-up.

All shifts are covered, and the work environment will most likely consist of an office or cubicle with a desk, computer, reference books, and, of course, a phone. Advice nurses can work for insurance companies, HMOs, PPOs, hospitals, or private companies who contract their services to any of the above. The pay has historically been slightly lower than hospital pay, but is becoming more competitive. It is an entirely different angle on patient care and can be a fun way to maintain contact with patients in a setting outside of the hospital.

Occasionally there are ads in the paper for this type of work. Another way to find positions is to contact insurance companies, HMOs, PPOs, and large hospital chains to find out if they offer telephone triage or advice lines. What you have to offer are your clinical and assessment skills, which are definitely transferable from the hospital to this setting.

▲ Sales

Companies that sell anything from IV systems and access products to pharmaceuticals often recognize the value of hiring nurses as sales representatives. Being a nurse provides you with immediate credibility, especially if you have used the product and can vouch for its effectiveness. Nurses speak the language of medical people, which is a great help in establishing a relationship based on trust and camaraderie. Nurses are also more likely to see how and where the product fits into the hospital's function, which gives them the edge on a non-medical person who may try to sell the hospital something they don't need. Organization, prioritization, the ability to do many things simultaneously, and communication skills are great assets in this field.

Cardiac monitors, IV pumps, specialty beds, IV systems, IV access devices, cardiac catheters, pacemakers, and defibrillators are just a few of the products that nurses are prime candidates to sell. Nurses have the necessary scientific knowledge and an understanding of human physiology and the disease process that is often required to work with the buyers *and* the end users (often other nurses). The sales rep could be calling on nurses, home health agencies, hospital purchasing departments, nurse managers and product utilization committee members, or even hospital administrators. When a sale involves equipment or products that will be utilized by nurses, the rep is often asked to train the staff on proper utilization and operation of the product. The sales rep who is also a nurse is often far more comfortable approaching nursing staff, better received by most nurses, able to anticipate questions and problems nurses may experience, and able to answer the inevitable clinical applications questions that arise during in-services.

Most sales reps work out of their homes and enjoy a flexible schedule. Time is spent in the home office on the phone making "cold calls," setting up appointments, and doing the ever-important follow-up on existing business. This field requires people who are highly motivated, since a great deal of time is spent in the field meeting with prospective customers. There can be a lot of rejection involved, but after the first few times of hurt feelings most reps learn to take it in stride, understand that it is part of the job, and do not take it personally. After a while, most reps build their reputation with a circle of solid clients and develop relationships of mutual trust, respect, and appreciation.

This job requires people who are energetic, motivated, self-starters willing to take a risk. It usually requires an initial cut in pay until commissions start to come in, after which many salespeople earn up to six figures! The salesperson must enjoy working independently, be willing to travel, and be flexible. A company car is often provided, along with an expense account for phone, travel, office supplies, meals, and entertainment.

A good way to identify a company that you may be interested in working for is to look around at work and identify your favorite products. It could be a cardiac monitor, an IV catheter, or even the brand of gloves that finally keeps your hands from getting chapped. Contacting these companies directly (your first cold call!) is usually a possibility. Or talk with your hospital's purchasing department—they may be able to provide you with names of reps for various companies or put you in contact with a rep they know well.

One nurse I spoke with recently went to a convention for urologists in San Francisco—not to see the urologists, but to visit the vendors booths that are a fixture at any convention. She took along some résumés and business cards, schmoozed a little, and passed her information on to the reps running the booths. She later got calls from five of the companies she contacted that day!

It can be exciting to be involved in the sale of a product that you have used and that you like. It can also be a terrific challenge to be involved in new products and cutting-edge technology as it emerges in the medical market. Companies are often willing to hire nurses without prior sales experience. Nurses are some of the most successful medical sales reps in the country!

▲ In-service education and training

If you are the type of person who likes the independence and travel associated with sales but not the pressures involved, there are still options for you. Most companies that sell technical products and equipment to hospitals have begun to utilize nurses to provide sales support in the in-servicing and training aspect of implementing a new product. You may work as an independent contractor or as an employee of the company. Either way, the pay is generally equal to or slightly higher than hospital pay, and all of your travel expenses are covered by the company. Some companies have had tremendous success in their clinical programs. One large hospital supply corporation has seen the ranks of its nurse consultants grow to 133 nurses in just four years!

Many hospitals are beginning to demand that companies provide clinical experts to train their staff. Compared to reps without a medical background, nurses are much more likely to succeed at answering clinical questions that arise in relation to implementing the product or equipment. They are able to establish rapport with hospital staff and troubleshoot problems as they arise. In these days of constant product changes, as prices fluctuate and new "deals" are signed, it has become even more essential for staff nurses to receive adequate training on the equipment they use. Many hospitals have an annual skills check-off, during which nurses must demonstrate their competency in the use of hospital equipment. Proper in-servicing has become more important than ever!

This job usually requires travel, is fast-paced and demanding. It provides a great deal of variety (especially if you can provide training on more than one product) and freedom in scheduling your time. It requires a positive, professional demeanor, as you are representing a company and can have an impact on their credibility. Flexibility is a must; scheduling and coordinating in-services is a real challenge, as last-minute schedule changes are common.

As discussed earlier in the section on sales, a good way to decide which companies you would like to work for is to pay attention to which products you enjoy using. A call to the company's education department can often put you in touch with the appropriate people to talk to. Five years ago, when I entered this field, my contact was made through a sales rep who came to do an in-service on a new product. (He was one of the few reps I didn't run and hide from!) We got to chatting, and I discovered that his company was just beginning a clinical program utilizing nurses to assist in product training. After a quick meeting a few days later in which we went over my experience and résumé, he made some calls, I was hired as a contractor, and the rest is history!

▲ Nurse consulting

It seems like "consulting" has become the new buzzword for the '90s, and that anyone with any skill whatsoever can print up business cards and call themselves a consultant. While this may be at least partly true, the fact is that these people provide a great service to companies that have trimmed their in-house resources to meet budgetary demands. For example, many hospitals don't feel they need a full-time employee to handle something like JCAHO surveys. But come survey time, they definitely need someone to ensure compliance and generally spiff up the place and prepare the staff. A nurse consultant might be able to do this job for them, then move on to the next job—thereby not requiring the hospital to have a full-time, benefited position.

The success of your consulting endeavors will largely depend on your proficiency in the area of your consulting expertise. Generally, you need strong clinical, theoretical, and administrative skills, in addition to a sharp mind and the ability to think on your feet and problem-solve almost anything. Fees vary widely, and may be charged by the hour, by the day, or by the project.

There are many companies that employ nurse consultants to do everything from cost containment studies to restructuring and change management. Nurses can assist health care providers and businesses in setting up and marketing new programs or services. Some companies hire nurse consultants to offer programs on health and wellness promotion, safety and accident prevention, stress reduction, and communication. A nurse consultant could also provide pre-employment physicals or drug testing for a company that doesn't have an in-house nurse. Look in your local phone book or call some of the local hospitals or businesses and ask them when and why they may have used nurse consultants. A little research at the library can provide you with a list of names of consulting agencies or businesses that may require the services of a consultant—just ask the reference librarian to help you.

Once you identify specific areas of specialty, businesses, or agencies you are interested in, you can then contact them, let them know what you have to offer, and see if your skills meet their needs. Consulting can be a pretty cutthroat industry. It is not unusual to run across highly competitive people who fear that your success could mean their failure. On the other hand, the free-spirited, explorative attitudes of many consultants can be like a breath of fresh air.

Another option is to position yourself as a consultant or independent contractor in any one of the many arenas that demand the occasional expertise of a nurse. Group homes for the mentally retarded and/or disabled, day care centers, and elder care centers, for example, will occasionally need on-site inspections or services. A nurse could provide home services to the families of newborns: newborn assessment, home bilirubin treatment, childproofing and other safety recommendations, lactation consulting, or childbirth education. Nurses are prime candidates for providing services to pain management centers, biofeedback and stress control clinics, and holistic health practitioners. If you can identify a niche that needs to be filled, *go for it!* Consulting is something you can do part-time, gradually building your business as you meet your monthly expenses in a regular part- or full-time job.

▲ *Medical-legal nurse consultant*

In a society as litigious as ours, is it any wonder that the field of medical-legal nurse consulting is expanding rapidly? Membership in the American Association of Legal Nurse Consultants (AALNC) grew from 35 in 1989 to 1,900 in 1996! Nurses are a valuable resource to attorneys in medical litigation. Attorneys and paralegals know all there is to know about most legal matters but do not generally have the expertise to deal with litigation in the area of medicine. Medical-legal nurse consultants work with lawyers in cases involving medical malpractice, litigation, personal injury, product liability, workers' comp, and criminal cases, among others. Nurses help the attorneys prepare their strategy, save them time by gathering information on the case, and then prepare the attorneys so that the medical information rolls off their tongues as easily as the "legal-ese" they normally speak.

Nurses may work for the plaintiff or the defense, ferreting out information that pertains to the case from patient's and doctor's records. Medical-legal nurse consultants can be instrumental in helping attorneys determine if they even *have* a case, especially in areas like personal injury. They are often asked to prepare a chronology of the case, determining the timeline of events and discovering any deviations from the standard of care that may have occurred.

This work requires research abilities, good teaching skills (a key element of the work is educating the attorneys), the ability to find appropriate medical professionals to act as expert witnesses, and availability to attend frequent meetings, trials, and depositions. You must possess excellent communication skills, the ability to write clear documents, and know how to present yourself in an appropriate manner. Educational background in law is not essential—your area of expertise is in the medical, not the legal, arena.

Legal nurse consultants can make from $50 to $100 per hour and up. They can work full- or part-time as independent contractors to a legal firm (or firms), full- or part-time as employees with a law firm, or even full- or part-time with an insurance company or hospital risk management department.

Breaking into this field may take some time. It can be done in conjunction with part-time work elsewhere. There are many seminars and workshops offered nationwide to prepare nurses to enter the field of medical legal consulting. Check the resource guide in this book for companies that provide training in this area. Through the use of videotaped presentations, you can study to become a consultant without ever leaving home! Once you are prepared, it's mainly a matter of marketing yourself to various law firms, then developing a reputation and working relationship with practicing attorneys. Once you're established, you may find that you can do this work full-time!

▲ Nursing instructor

Teaching in a nursing school is a possibility even if you don't have a graduate degree. Working in this setting allows you to polish your skills and knowledge of clinical nursing and sharpen your skills as you supervise novice nurses in the clinical setting. It is a terrific opportunity to act as a mentor and role model. We probably all have a particular nursing instructor who had a huge impact on how we felt about nursing and our ability to be a "good nurse." The academic world of nursing is a lot different than the "real world." It has to be. The foundation upon which the new nurse builds her clinical skills is laid in this setting. You will probably encounter some strong suggestions (read: *pressure*) to advance your education if you work in higher education for any length of time, and the expectation often exists that you write (and publish) articles and participate in programs to advance your learning.

Although most educational institutions require an MSN and recent clinical experience, some ADN, LVN, and CNA programs will still hire a nurse with a BSN. Pay in this setting is frequently not as high as hospital nursing, but there are some definite perks—such as no night shifts, and weekends, holidays, and summers off! Many instructors find the work very rewarding and cherish their roles as mentor to new nurses. Nursing instructors who emphasize empowerment of their students can leave a lasting impression.

▲ Entrepreneurship

If you are a nurse who has an interest in developing your own business, *run*, do not walk, to the nearest Small Business Development Association (SBDA) and make an appointment to see one of their counselors. There are more than 750 SBDAs nationwide, and the services they offer are *free!* (Well, not exactly free, because they are a branch of the U.S. Small Business Administration and operate with our tax dollars.)

The SBDAs are designed to support you through the process of starting a business or expanding an existing business. They have a wealth of information and services and sponsor SCORE (Service Corps of Retired Executives), a group of retired businesspeople with whom you can meet in one-on-one counseling sessions. These people can assist you in writing a business and/or marketing plan, securing finances, and obtaining necessary business licenses, permits, and insurance. This organization is a *tremendous* resource and contributes greatly to the success of small businesses in a world where the failure rate is more than 50% within the first five years.

Another essential resource for the nurse entrepreneur is the book, *Entrepreneuring: A Nurse's Guide to Starting a Business,* by Gerry Vogel and Nancy Doleysh. Specifically geared toward nurses, this book guides you through the process of determining if your personality is that of an entrepreneur, then finding a niche and establishing a business, and marketing and financing that business. It offers invaluable insight on what it takes to succeed in this exciting and challenging career choice.

Starting your own business can be one of the most challenging and rewarding experiences of your life. It is also likely to be more work than you can imagine. Make sure that you have the skills you need to make the business work, a service or product that is wanted and needed by the public, access to enough money to get started, and a solid business and marketing plan. Even with all of these factors in place, a new small business has a relatively low chance of success. My belief is that success in this arena comes from starting a business that involves something you *love* to do (believe me—you'll be doing it a lot!), learning to be extremely flexible, and being as tenacious as a pit bull. The right combination of passion, flexibility, and tenacity is a bottom-line requirement for a successful entrepreneur.

CHAPTER 5

Mentorship

Now that you have gained some insight into what you like to do and what you *want* to do, and have examined some of the options that exist for nurses, it's time to take a serious look at how to put all of this information to use. One of the most effective ways of moving from the assessment or discovery stage through the planning stage to the realization of your dreams is asking for help. For centuries upon centuries, novices have sought out the advice and vision of experts.

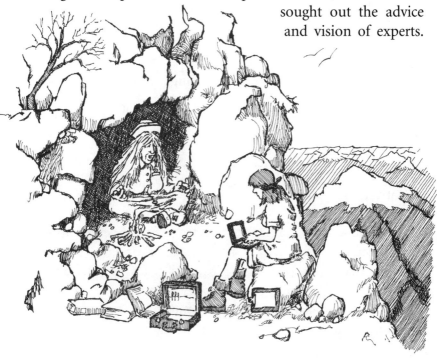

Whether it's a young person seeking the "truth" from a guru on a mountaintop or a middle-aged nurse seeking guidance from a wise and experienced person who has already walked a similar path, this type of mentorship has, again and again, proven to be of value for those choosing to make changes in their life.

The word *mentor* is adapted from Greek mythology; it means an experienced guide, adviser, or advocate who assumes responsibility for promoting the growth and professional advancement of a less experienced individual—the *protégé*. This type of mentoring has been common in the business world for ages. Successful, well-established professionals agree to provide long-term guidance to aid career development of newcomers.

Mentoring relationships have also been well utilized by nurses in administrative and academic positions. According to C. Vance in "Women Leaders: Modern-day Heroines or Societal Deviants?" (an article written for *Image* magazine in 1979), mentors have helped novice nurses through:

1. Career promotion, door opening, and creating opportunities;

2. Professional career role-modeling;

3. Intellectual and scholarly stimulation; and

4. Inspiration.

Of the *mentees* in this article, 93% went on to serve as mentors to others—a clear statement as to the value these nurses placed on the experience.

Staff nurses have tended to perform a similar service to less experienced nurses (such as new grads or orientees) in the form of orientation, preceptorships, and coaching. These tend to be short-term arrangements to facilitate not only staff orientation, but also socialization of newcomers. As a preceptor, you function as an intense, one-on-one educator and role model for students, new grads, or new staff. As a coach, you may be asked to assist less experienced co-workers in determining their special needs for clinical growth, help them set goals, assign tasks to challenge them and improve their skills, and provide feedback on their performance and goal achievement.

Some hospitals consistently use these types of programs. Others do not. Consequently, there has not been a consistent practice of mentoring within the nursing profession. This may be due to a variety of factors, such as lack of exposure to the concept, minimal participation in team sports as children, lack of self-esteem, lack of socialization towards affiliation, or absence of a career orientation.

Traditional mentoring programs certainly have a proven track record. However, it's possible that the type of mentoring that has been so successful in the business world may not meet the needs of nurses. Nurses have different values and expectations in the educational and service arenas than businesspeople do. Therefore, the "business formula" probably cannot become the "nursing formula." Also, nurses have a long history of being infinitely more compassionate and helpful to their patients than to their co-workers. I remember reading an article years ago called "Do Nurses Really Eat Their Young?" I was shocked and slightly resentful of the title, but as I read the article, bits of insight into the nursing profession began to creep into my mind. That insight, combined with years of experience in many different hospitals, has confirmed that there is a tendency for "old timers" to stereotype new grads, distrust the novices' technical competence, and even resent the newcomers' enthusiasm and attempts to institute change. Of course, *you* would never do this! But have you ever seen nurses with these tendencies?

This makes me think about when my career took a shift from ICU to L&D. Much to my surprise, this was an *extremely* difficult transition. After seven years of experience as an ICU nurse, when I moved into L&D I was suddenly treated as if I knew nothing. Now, I didn't expect to walk into an entirely new area of nursing and know everything, but we're talking basics here. Even though caring for laboring patients is radically different than caring for critically ill patients, my clinical skills were sound. My ability to understand the unspoken rules of the game, however, was sadly lacking. It seemed as if an entirely different type of teamwork, with an entirely different set of rules, existed in labor and delivery. I was well versed at functioning as a member of an ICU team, but quite unprepared to meet the unspoken expectations of this new environment. Rather than appreciating the differences and valuing what I did have to offer, the general attitude toward me seemed to be mistrust, resentment, and judgment. This experience was shocking after being an accepted team member in critical care nursing for so many years. I didn't expect it. This type of thing only happens to new grads, right?

On the other hand, I've encountered several nurses during my career who had a deep and memorable impact, not only on my ability to become expert at my work, but also on my personal growth and sense of self. They did this by functioning as role models. It was unspoken and unplanned, but very effective. Imagine if we all had an agreement with someone who would listen to us and provide us with feedback, insight, and advice based on their experience. Having a mentor during my transition from ICU to labor and delivery might have alerted me to the complex problems I was facing long before I was able to figure things out on my own.

Dr. Linda Phillips-Jones, an extremely gifted psychologist and mentoring consultant for some of the largest corporations in this country, wrote a book, *The New Mentors and Protégés: How to Succeed with the New Mentoring Partnerships*. In it, she describes mentors as "influential, experienced people who personally help you reach your major life goals ... Finding and making use of the right mentors is the most critical step you'll ever take in your career." Notice she said *mentors*—plural. In her research, she found that the "new protégés" have figured out that investing energy in one mentor isn't wise; in fact, it's naive to expect one person to provide everything. Many protégés are acquiring two or more mentors to help them work on different goals, and they know their mentoring relationships are likely to be shorter than the relationships of the past.

Dr. Phillips-Jones goes on to say: "During the past twelve years, the typical length and focus of mentoring relationships has taken a noticeable turn. The new mentors and protégés are very pragmatic. Relationships, even the 'informal' ones that evolve outside of organizations, are more structured than they used to be ... Parameters are set, goals are outlined, and a relatively short timeframe for the relationships is proposed. Most pairs propose working together for weeks or months, almost never for years."

This kind of mentorship relationship seems like a better "fit" with nursing than traditional business models for several reasons. In a profession that does not have a long history of mentoring or understanding of the etiquette involved, it seems more reasonable to focus on short-term goals rather than long-term goals in terms of the mentoring relationship. This arrangement is less threatening or intimidating, since it allows you to dip your toe into the water rather than feel forced to plug your nose and dive in. It also closely parallels the structures already familiar to most nurses: precepting, orienting, and coaching. Only this time the focus is on *you*. Big difference!

So, in what ways would it benefit you to work with a mentor? Dr. Phillips-Jones describes the advantages of entering into mentor/mentee relationships as multi-faceted. Mentors can provide you with advice and help you set some definite career and life goals. They can give you encouragement, often cited by people who have achieved success as the most valuable help they ever received. Changing your career and your life can be extremely difficult, and it is not unusual to get discouraged and lose hope. Having someone to share their ups and downs with you can be the boost that you need to keep going. Mentors can teach you new skills and improve your knowledge. A glance at history will provide many examples of masters passing their knowledge on to apprentices. Mentors can be a model for you to follow. You can examine their stories and life experiences to see how someone else handled a situation that may be particularly baffling or scary. Then you can decide whether to copy the behavior, dismiss it, or use their method as a base with which you can blend your own ideas.

Mentors provide mentees with opportunities and resources. Maybe you have been dying to meet the nurse who opened her own business in medical transcription, and your mentor is a friend of a friend. Often, mentors are more aware of resources and can help you find your way through the library, advise you on the most appropriate professional organizations, or locate members of the community who can assist you. Mentors can increase your exposure and visibility by putting you in front of the right people. Don't underestimate the value of your mentor's endorsement—your ideas are much more likely to be accepted and noticed if they're promoted or even casually mentioned by someone important. Finally, mentors can provide you with a bridge to maturity. Their guidance and example can be the bridge over troubled waters that symbolizes the difficult transitions in your life.

Sounds good, huh? But ... now the excuses come. You don't want to take up someone's time. What if the relationship doesn't work out? You hate it when someone gives you advice. You don't know who you would ask to be a mentor. It all seems like too much of a bother. You can make it on your own, thank you very much … and on and on. The fact is, it is *always* your choice, and you decide which tools *you* want to use on your road to career development. However, please don't underestimate the potential that exists in the mentor/mentee relationship. Let's dispel some myths:

1. *You don't want to take up someone's time.*

Rest assured that mentoring is a two-way exchange, and your mentor also benefits enormously from your relationship — sometimes far more than you do. Have you ever had the opportunity to be a guiding influence in someone else's life? Maybe at work, as a preceptor. Or at home, with your children. Or maybe with a little sister or brother, or friend.

People mentor others for lots of reasons. Perhaps someone helped them at a time when they felt lost and stuck, and, with the help of the mentor, they were finally able to achieve their dream. Maybe you remind them of someone they once knew and weren't able to help at the time. Or their intuition tells them they want to help you. Or your project closely parallels their own dream and allows them to vicariously experience the joy of completion through you. Maybe they admire you, your goals, and your vision. Maybe they just like to cheer for the underdog. Their reasons stem from a variety of sources, including past experiences in these kinds of relationships, self-image, and basic values, goals, and needs. The mentoring relationship can provide fulfillment to all parties involved, though probably for vastly different reasons.

2. *What if the relationship doesn't work out?*

If you do your "front work" carefully and with a lot of thought, you can avoid some of the major pitfalls that can occur in the mentor/mentee relationship. Dr. Phillips-Jones describes this front work as "the right formula."

The first ingredient in the formula is *mutual respect*. Respect and trust are essential for successful relationships. You have to truly believe that your mentor has enough status, skill, or power to help you before you'll accept them in that role. At the same time, your mentor must have a positive attitude about you and feel that you'd be a good investment, worth the time and energy it would take to groom you. It is important to talk about your expectations for the mentoring relationship up front to make sure that you are both on the same track. Finding a good match in terms of goals and expectations is an excellent start.

The second ingredient is to determine the *appropriate quantity and quality of mentoring*. If you do not see the assistance offered as appropriate or valuable to you, or if you find the information outdated, superficial, or not worth the time and energy, chances are the mentoring relationship will not work. Remember, though, sometimes things that don't feel quite right at the moment turn out to be incredibly valuable in the long-run. Don't let your resistance, judgment, or preconceived notions keep you from seeing the value of the help offered. Sometimes a tough call to make, but simply keeping an open mind goes a long way.

The third and last ingredient is *proper timing*. Whether or not mentoring will work depends on where you *and* your mentor are in your own lives, plus the specific timing of your initial contact. It is not unusual to look at an opportunity you may have strolled right past three years ago and wish it would come along now, when you really need it and are ready for it.

3.   *You don't know who you would ask to be your mentor.*

If you are like most potential protégés, you probably don't personally know any mentors who could provide the help you want. And even if you do know someone, you might not know how to approach them. Again, if we turn to Dr. Phillips-Jones and follow her suggestions, a seemingly impossible task is made simple.

First, identify what (not *who*) you need. Make a list of the kind of help you'd like to have. Ask yourself: If you were as successful as you wanted to be right now, what would be happening? Would you be learning new skills, getting financial backing for your ideas, or finding out how to plan and implement a project? Perhaps trying out a new lifestyle, or writing and publishing an article or book? Earning more money? Starting a new job? Getting feedback on your style, appearance, or progress? Careful thought should go into making this list for two reasons: (1) perhaps some of your needs can be met by other resources besides mentors, and (2) the list will help you be very clear about what you're asking for when the time comes. Make it easy for your mentors to meet your needs by presenting your goals in a specific and logical way.

Next, evaluate yourself as a prospective mentee. Are you open to receiving help from others? How do you really feel about becoming a mentee? How "dependent" are you willing to become? How can you maintain that balance between dependence and independence that you've worked so hard to attain? Are you willing and able to ask someone for help? Is it difficult for you to be in the receiving role instead of the giving role? If you see potential problems here, it may mean that you need to find a mentor who would prefer to play a more passive role in the relationship. Or you can experiment with the more traditional approach to mentorship and see what happens if you make some custom-made modifications. It may not be as hard as you think. Remember, it's only temporary.

Now, identify some mentor candidates. Go through your list of needs once again. Begin to make a list of some possible mentors. You may want to list more than one person for a particular need. Use your imagination and think of anyone who might be able to help you in your endeavor. Think about the most influential people you know, who might be able to help you directly or know someone who could. Who do you know that thinks you have potential? Who has recently achieved the things you want and might be inspired to help you? Who has helped you in the past and might help again?

Maybe you're thinking of a few people who seem like they would make good mentors, but you can't identify exactly what they could do for you at this point. Put them on your list anyway, and see if you can learn more about them. Something about them might surface that will present a new aspect of potential help to you.

As you look at your completed list, begin to ask yourself some questions about each candidate: Where are the potential mentors in terms of their own careers? Are they just beginning, or are they perhaps switching career fields? How influential are they? Do they hold any offices, or have they received any honors? What is their current situation? Are they in the middle of a crisis? Put yourself in their shoes and ask if you would be ready to help someone else at this particular time. If they're under a lot of pressure, that could possibly lead to negative consequences for you. Have these potential mentors ever helped others? In what ways? How do they feel about mentoring? Can you talk to their former protégés? Bear in mind that even though these potential mentors might not have helped others, they may still be able to help you. Perhaps no one has ever requested their assistance before.

If you already know the possible mentor, evaluate your relationship with them. Would adding the mentor-mentee dimension have a positive or negative effect? Do you share similar goals and values? If the potential mentor is very different from you but can be of great help, try to figure out ways to work around or at least tolerate the differences for as long as the relationship is valuable.

Before you approach your candidate, do some preparation. Find out all you can about the individual's work, special interests, and needs. Talk to others who know them. Overall, think through your request before you present it. Anticipate every possible question or negative response and have answers for each. Once you've anticipated all of the obstacles and thought through some creative ways around them, you're ready to take the plunge.

After all this preparation, the time has come to approach your possible mentors. Common sense and courtesy can be your guide here. Probably the oldest (and safest) way to make the initial contact is to ask a mutual acquaintance to mention you to the potential mentor. Ask them to put in a good word for you—don't hesitate to capitalize on the power of a referral! Just be certain that your mutual acquaintance sees you as favorably as you think they do. If you're not sure, ask them for a frank reaction.

This is the approach I used to initiate the mentoring relationship that helped me write this book. My good friend Marti was in a graduate nursing program and raved constantly about one of her professors. Everything I heard about this professor told me that our values were similar, and she'd been in nursing for over 35 years! She'd had lots of exposure to student nurses, people in transition, and nurses in the midst of a major career shift. I asked Marti to approach the professor to see if she was interested in establishing a mentor/mentee relationship with me. Once this initial step had been taken, I simply called at the agreed-upon time, explained who I was and what I hoped to accomplish, and *asked for her help.*

When such contacts aren't possible, many people simply "put their cards on the table" and write the person a letter. Try to compliment the person on something they've done, and then share something about yourself that will spark some interest. If you can think of anything that you might be able to do for them, by all means mention it. If your request relates to a project, include examples of your work, if possible.

Once you've arranged a meeting with your possible mentor, be sure to do your homework before you get there. Decide on your personal agenda, and what you want the meeting's outcome to be. Be sure you are clear about your needs, your goals, and your vision. Respect is being established here, so take care to dress appropriately and decide in advance what you'll say—and what you won't say. During the meeting, listen attentively, show interest in any concerns, and agree to consider any advice you're given. Be specific in your request for help.

Follow up the meeting with an appreciative note or phone call. Tell your mentor how much the visit meant to you, and comment on a specific thing they said to you, if possible.

If your request didn't work out, analyze why it failed. Did you ask for too much? How was your timing? Did you select the wrong person? Did you clarify exactly what you wanted? Did you remember to think of ways to make the experience beneficial for the other person? Did you come on too strong? Could you have been the five-hundredth person that day to ask for something?

If you think there was some glimmer of a chance with this person, you can try another approach, or maybe wait a few weeks and make contact again. But if it was a definite no-go and feels like a lost cause, move on to the next person as soon as possible. The proverbial "getting back up on the horse" definitely applies here. Don't let yourself be scared away because of one attempt that didn't click. Before you know it, you'll find yourself right smack in the middle of a mentoring relationship!

These steps can be of great value on your path to developing successful mentoring relationships. Evaluate the goals you've established and see if there are any areas in which a mentor could assist you. Maybe a mentor could help you to clarify your goals or work toward making them more specific. They might provide guidance and feedback as you go through the processes of developing your résumé, interviewing, and deciding on job offers.

This process can feel scary for nurses. We have not, traditionally, been oriented toward finding out what can help meet *our* needs and goals. I have to admit that I was a nervous wreck when I made the initial phone call to a potential mentor. However, one thing I have learned in the past few years, that has proven to be true again and again, is that if I feel afraid or resistant to try something new, it is usually related to not being familiar with it, not feeling good enough about myself to do it, or being afraid I'll fall flat on my face. What I've also found to be true is that the only way to *get* familiar with something new is to *try it*, that we are *ALL* good enough, and that life goes on after a few scratches on the nose!

If you have an interest in the mentor-mentee relationship, want to seek out a mentor, or even want to *be* a mentor, I would definitely recommend reading Linda Phillips-Jones' *The New Mentors and Protégés*. Or, you may want to obtain Dr. Phillips-Jones' *The Mentoring Program Design Package*. It contains a coordinator's guide, mentor's guide, and mentee's guide — everything you would need to set up a mentoring program in your workplace. You can order either or both of these resources from:

Coalition of Counseling Centers
13560 Mesa Drive
Grass Valley, CA 95949
916-268-1146

CHAPTER 6

Planning Your Future

It has been said that a goal is "a dream with a deadline." To dream is to imagine or visualize something that may not exist for you now, but that you would like to have be a part of your life. We all have some things that are "left undone" in our lives, still in the "dream" phase. Things you are going to do ... *someday*. You know what it is that you want, and maybe even what it would take to get there, but you just haven't taken the time to get specific and make it a goal. A good place to start when planning your future is to answer the question: "Someday I'm going to ..." and list as many ideas as come into your mind.

Answering this question can give you some idea of areas in your life that need attention and can provide a basis for goal-setting. To set goals is to get specific with your dreams and pull them into a format that is made up of concrete, achievable steps. Following these steps puts you on a path to making your dreams into reality.

A few years ago a nationwide survey was conducted in America about goal setting. Results of the study showed that only about 3% of people surveyed had written plans or goals for life. An additional 10% reported having goals or a fairly good idea about their life objectives, but hadn't written them down. Another 60% had some idea of what they needed financially to retire in some reasonable fashion, but that was about it. More than 25% said they hadn't given any significant thought to goals or future planning at all. Interestingly, 3% were considered highly successful, 10% were considered comfortable, 60% were of modest means, and about 30% were struggling in life (Winwood, 1990).

Nurses are not strangers to the importance and effectiveness of setting long- and short-term goals. You do this all the time for your patients, whether it takes the form of a care plan, a clinical pathway, or merely something you do in your head. Maybe it is just because you have a written tool that acts as a gauge and spurs on your activity. Or maybe it is just the process of focusing your thinking and clarifying priorities. But there is little doubt that well-planned and well-implemented care leads to more positive outcomes.

Once again, you are being asked to turn this process inward. Be as thorough and careful with your plan for yourself as you would be for your patients. Some points to remember as you develop your goals are:

▲ Write your goals down. They can then be used as a gauge to measure your progress. This lends a feeling of commitment and purpose to your work, and allows you to review your goals periodically for motivation and bragging!

▲ Ensure that your goals are motivated by your values. As mentioned earlier, if you experience a gap between your values and your daily actions, this can be an indication that developing a goal in this area would help you achieve your dreams.

▲ Goals should be clear and specific. The more clearly you define your desired outcome, the more specifically you will be able to focus your thinking and develop an achievable plan.

▲ Goals should be measurable and time-related.
A deadline provides you with a sense of urgency
to act and serves as an external reminder of your
internal commitment.

▲ Goals should be personal and attainable. Your goals
are developed from your values, which arise out of
your inner self. Goals make you reach, stretch, and
change, but they must be within your grasp or they
simply set you up for failure.

Given all that information, now you are fully prepared to
write down your goals, right? Getting started in goal-setting is
much like learning any new skill—sometimes it helps to have
examples and other triggers to get you thinking about appropriate goals for your life. The following list of categories represents the most common areas of goal-setting. You may want to
add your own categories. These are simply some ideas and a
place to start.

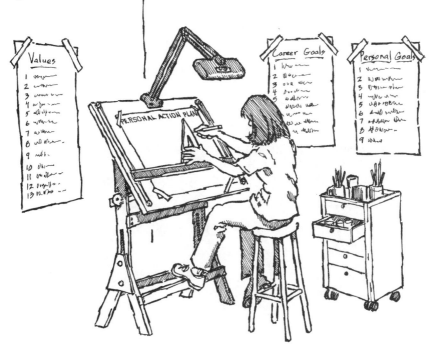

PHYSICAL

- ▲ Have I had a complete medical/dental examination in the last year?

- ▲ Do I exercise regularly?

- ▲ Am I at my optimum weight level?

- ▲ Do I have any destructive habits that need control?

FAMILY

- ▲ Am I spending enough quality time with my family?

- ▲ Do I spend enough time by myself, doing what I need/want to do?

- ▲ Do I spend one-on-one time with each of my children?

- ▲ Do I help plan family activities? Family vacations?

- ▲ Have I taken a vacation recently?

- ▲ Do I take my work home frequently?

SPIRITUAL / HUMANITARIAN

- ▲ Have I volunteered to help another in need lately?

- ▲ Am I living according to my moral and ethical principles?

- ▲ Do I attend spiritual gatherings, such as church, temple, or meetings?

- ▲ Do I project a teachable, approachable, and humble attitude?

CAREER

- ▲ Am I happy doing the work I currently do?

- ▲ Do I have a plan for career development?

- ▲ Do I understand my goals for development and how to get there?

- ▲ Have I communicated my expectations to my family, friends, and/or boss?

- ▲ Is there any way I can be more effective on the job?

- ▲ Am I contributing to the growth and development of my peers and subordinates?

FINANCIAL

- ▲ Am I living within my income?

- ▲ Do I have an ongoing savings or investment plan?

- ▲ Will I have the money I need to retire in the timeframe I want to?

- ▲ Am I using credit wisely?

COMMUNITY / POLITICAL

- ▲ Am I aware of and helping solve community problems?

- ▲ Do I actively support my political party? Are political causes important to me?

- ▲ Am I engaged in positive community causes?

- ▲ Are my neighbors known to me and I to them?

EDUCATIONAL / PERSONAL DEVELOPMENT

▲ Is my education and training well rounded?

▲ Do I have a reading list of subjects to learn about?

▲ Have I been to the theater, art show, or concert lately?

▲ Have I planned time for rest and recreation?

These questions are designed to trigger some ideas for goals and to test your emotional response to each category. Because there may be a higher level of urgency to work on an item that makes you feel the most uncomfortable, start with the item that, according to your conscience, needs the most attention.

Write your goals in the same way you would write your patient's goals, but instead of writing something like, "Patient will return to full independent function post–total knee replacement," you might write, "In two years, I will have completed a college-level course in watercolor painting." Refer to your core values, identified in exercise 2, Chapter 3. Write a long-term goal for each of the values you feel is a priority. Try not to be overwhelmed at this point if you have several long-term goals.

You may use the form on page 105, which I developed for the class, Managing Change, in 1994, as a guideline. Write your value statement at the top of the page, followed by your long-term goal. Use as many pages as you need; each long-term goal gets a page. These pages will become your personal action plan.

You can also make up your own form or utilize one of the many planning systems available on the market. A list of recommended systems and where you can get them is given in the resource guide at the end of this book.

Once you've written out your long-term goals, break them down and determine what the major steps would be to accom-

	Personal Action Plan	
Value: _____		
Long-Term Goal: _____		
Short-Term Goal: _____		

✓	Daily Tasks	Deadline

plish each goal. These are your short-term goals. For example, if your value had to do with appreciating art and your long-term goal was to take some art classes, then a good short-term goal could be to take a college-level course in watercolor painting. Now, break it down even further into the actual tasks that need to be completed. You might want to list tasks related to determining which colleges offer art courses, what the schedule is, how much it would cost, budgeting time and money to enable you to take the course, registering for the course ... See how this works? In this way, the dream of learning to paint with watercolors can become a reality.

Nurses are actually at an advantage here. We know how to plan. For the patient mentioned a minute ago, whose long-term goal was to return to full independent function following knee surgery, a short-term goal might be: "Patient will be able to ambulate independently by post-operative day (POD) #3." We could then break this down into tasks such as teaching post-operative isometric exercises, contacting PT to train patient on crutches, dangle patient at bedside on POD #1, up in chair by POD #2 ... See? We've all done this a million times for others. Now, it's your turn to plan for *you!*

When you plan your month, or your week, or your day, you can refer to these pages to determine what needs to be done by what date in order for you to achieve your goal. This process, which may seem a little cumbersome at first, has been invaluable to me. For instance, when I first decided to write this book, about three years ago, the task seemed daunting. I figured if I could just get an outline done, then I would be off and running, quite sure of what to do next. Once the outline was done, I found myself even *more* overwhelmed. There was so much to do, it seemed I would never get it all done. So, the outline got pared down and more specific. This helped, but it only addressed what needed to be *written*, not everything that needed to be *done*.

When I decided to apply the principles I'd learned for career development, things really began to get clear. My long-term goal (to help bring quality works of writing into the world to benefit nurses and others) and short-term goal (to write and publish a book on career development for nurses) were already clear. I pored over all of my books on writing and publishing and pulled out all of the tasks that needed to be done. It took days to complete this list, prioritize it, and make sure that all of the deadlines involved in publishing were in the right place. It took a lot of guessing, too—I had to be willing to just *make up* some dates. For example, determining when the rough draft would be completed (who knew?). Then I broke the prioritized list down into months and made a separate sheet for each month that contained the tasks to be done and their deadlines. I placed these sheets in my Franklin planner and referred to them almost daily as I worked toward completion of the task-that-seemed-impossible. I can't tell you how great it felt to check things off, one by one, knowing I was actually achieving a dream of mine! Without those lists, I'm not sure I ever would have gotten past the "Someday I'm going to …" stage. It really works and is worth every ounce of effort you put into it!

Implementation

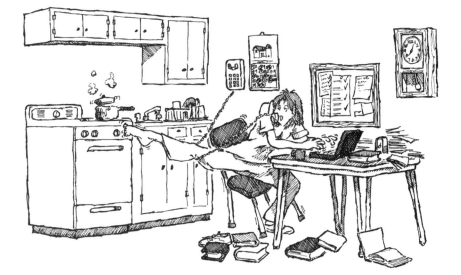

CHAPTER 7

Bringing It All Together

Before digging into preparing cover letters, résumés, interviewing, and thank-you letters, take some time to do a quick summary of all that you have accomplished to this point. If you have followed the steps outlined in the prior chapters, then you have:

▲ Identified those skills that you most enjoy and examined their transferability to other settings

▲ Examined current career options for nurses

▲ Elicited support by contacting a mentor or asking friends, family, and/or peers to act as your coach

▲ Identified your values and goals

▲ Formulated your personal action plan

Whew! This is a tremendous amount of work ... and it's a remarkable achievement. Keep in mind that only about 3% of Americans have written goals or plans for their life! Take a moment here to congratulate yourself—reach around and pat yourself on the back. The value of the work you've done so far is, without question, enormous. This is information that can sharpen and clarify your sense of yourself in the world, and has applications both on and off the job.

THE "RULES OF THE GAME"

The next phase, in which all this hard work is pulled into a format that can create openings in the world of work, was a bit of a struggle for me personally. I talked about my own resistance earlier ... well, it went off the scale when I got to this point! Never one to enjoy what always seemed like "games" one is expected to play, I went into full-scale rebellion! All it took was someone suggesting that I be "proactive," and get out there to "network" to find the kind of work I wanted, and the muttering would begin. (Aaargh! The N-word! Since when is it acceptable English to use a noun as a verb? And just what the heck does "network" *mean*, anyway?) I had a mental image of all these plastic Barbie and Ken dolls in a room together, smiles plastered on their faces, robotically shaking hands and exchanging business cards. I'd rather die, I thought with firm resolution.

Well, with the loving support of my own mentors and peers, I was finally able to make peace with the "process" of bringing it all together. A friend recommended the book *How to Work a Room*, by Susan RoAne (which, by the way, is a readable—even enjoyable—book on the rules of the networking game). Another friend, Marti, helped me reframe the word "networking" by figuring out what it really meant for me. We had a good time coming up with alternatives for the N-word—like chatting, sharing, being friendly, flirting, and schmoozing. Now, when someone comes to me with the suggestion that I network, I can just substitute the appropriate word in my mind. I picked up another book, *Hardball for Women: Winning at the Game of Business* by Pat Heim, which was *very* enlightening. It helped me understand how all the rules of the game came to be in the first place, and offered insight into how the world of business is conducted as a sport. Women, especially, tend to be at a disadvantage until they can understand these rules and use them to get ahead. I really enjoyed this book, found it fascinating, and highly recommend it.

They say that information is power, and I have found this to be especially true when working in the arena of résumés, cover letters, and interviewing. Gaining a new perspective as to *why* it is so important to know the rules of the game helped me to make the choice *to play* the game—at least to some degree. At the very least, you can level the playing field somewhat (see —just like baseball!) by understanding the rules and how they apply to your setting.

Most nurses I've known are pretty much like me—they are not crazy about the idea of playing these types of games, never *had* to play games to get work, and don't *want* to have to play games to get work now. It was a huge struggle for me to write this chapter. Not because the information is so difficult or hard to understand. *Au contraire.* It's really quite simple. It was a struggle because it all seems so petty and unnecessary. I'd much rather be able to just sit down and talk to people, openly and honestly. Put it all on the table and come to an agreement, amen and hallelujah.

But the reality is that there *are* certain expected behaviors and rules of etiquette in the business world — *and* in the nursing world. The reality is that you are working with people of many different personalities and cultures who don't know you from Adam, and it is not always just as simple as sitting down for a heart-to-heart talk. Rules are generally in place for a reason. In this case, they seem to be important in that they allow you to talk to someone you've never met before, gather information, demonstrate capability, and secure employment that you love and enjoy. This, I've sadly come to realize, may not even be possible without at least *some* understanding of *the rules.*

The following information, and there is a lot of it, is my best attempt at presenting the rules of the game in a tailored-for-nurses format. There are many, many books out there on these topics that can be used to expand your understanding of these rules. Even if you choose to avoid the machinations that have come to be expected, it is *still* helpful to know what they are. Most people find their own "comfort zone" with information like this, much like I did. Some want to perform to a tee (and would probably *love* working in sales!), and others want to be able to scrape by on the barest minimum of such nonsense. Make no mistake here—it might seem like nonsense, but, to a certain degree, it has become the standard. It's really not so hard, and if you think of it as a game (which it really *is*), it can even be fun! So, let the games begin!

RÉSUMÉS

The hard work you have done to this point has given you the foundation you need to prepare a résumé that accurately reflects who you are, what you have to offer, and what you most love to do. In fact, each of the exercises you've completed play an important role in the development of a good résumé. Let's take a closer look:

▲ *Skills* (Chapter 3)

In today's working world, "skills = marketability." Becoming very clear about what your skills are allows you to focus your résumé on achievements that convey the very best of what you have to offer a prospective employer. This is, after all, what a résumé is: a tool for conveying what you have to offer to someone who is seeking to fill a need. A specifically targeted résumé based on your skills and achievements is more likely to demonstrate transferability to a prospective employer when you want to move into a new career area.

▲ *Options* (Chapter 4)

Becoming aware of all the options that exist for nursing professionals is a key step in identifying where you can find a "good match." A clear understanding of the options that most interest you allows you to set the tone for your résumé, and largely determines its content. Different arenas in health care have different cultures, and it is important to speak the language of the natives! Once your résumé is written, it will be important to get feedback from people within the "culture," in the form of informational interviews or assistance from your mentor, to ensure the appropriateness of your approach.

For example, imagine if someone approached a nurse manager who was seeking to hire a staff nurse for a med/surg unit with a résumé that was strictly tailored to the business world—achievement-based, results-oriented, and focused on skills that one would need to succeed in business. Would that applicant's résumé effectively convey the clinical skills, communication skills, and ability to work as a team member that are so important to the role of a staff nurse? By the same token, a nurse approaching the hiring manager in a large hospital supply corporation for a sales rep position is not going to project a compelling picture of the required capabilities if the résumé is focused on clinical skills, listing past hospital employment and a short description of the duties performed. Narrowing the field and targeting your audience is crucial to submitting a résumé that will stand out among the *many* that are received for most jobs.

▲ *Support/mentor* (Chapter 5)

Having a support person (or persons) can be helpful in the process of distilling the *vast* amount of information obtained in the earlier exercises into the little one-page document called a résumé. To do this effectively, you need someone who is the objective other—someone you can try out new ideas on and who will offer you feedback based on personal experience or their understanding of you and your values and goals. Your support person helps spur you on when the going gets tough, laughs with you when you take this whole process too seriously, provides an anchor for you when you get distracted, and holds your hand when things get overwhelming.

▲ *Values and goals* (Chapters 3 and 6)

To a large extent, the career option you choose is directed by your values and goals. These same values and goals are an underlying focus for your résumé. They are a measuring tool which can be utilized to ensure that your résumé reflects the entirety of *you*: your priorities, dreams, achievements, and, to some degree, your personality. It is important not to get *too* serious about writing the "perfect résumé." You could end up with a document that is tailored to the needs of the company but doesn't remotely express *you*. Stay focused on what *you* have to offer *them*. Frequently reviewing your values and goals in the process of writing your résumé allows you to create a more genuine representation of the big-picture you. After all, the goal here is to get the job you *want*, not just to get a job. Don't fall into the trap of losing sight of your values and goals in an attempt to become the "perfect candidate."

▲ *Personal action plan* (Chapter 6)

Your résumé is one of many tools that you use to achieve work-related goals reflected in your action plan. Working closely with your action plan in the process of preparing your résumé optimizes your ability to shift your career in a way that moves you toward completion of your stated goals.

▲ ▲ ▲

As you have probably guessed, it will be important for you to refer frequently to your responses from the exercises in the prior chapters—especially Chapters 3 and 6.

The nuts and bolts of writing résumés are covered in many, many books—some of which are truly great resources. What I have found, however, is that the nursing profession plays by a somewhat different set of rules than the business world, toward which many of the books are geared. As mentioned earlier, each work setting has its own culture. The same is true for professions. Can you identify any work culture differences between nursing and, say, engineering? Or accounting? Business? An approach considered tame in one culture could be considered pushy or overboard in another. So this chapter will focus on the development of a résumé that most clearly reflects *you*, targets a position that is a good match, and is geared toward your expected audience.

The overall purpose of your résumé is to summarize your personal achievements and employment experience. Your mission (should you decide to accept it) is to present this information in a way that makes you stand out from the crowd and clearly communicates your skills and your personal style to the company you are interested in. Even though there are many "recipes" out there, and lots of experts to tell you the best way to construct your résumé, even the *experts* don't all agree on what that best way is. Some people prefer a chronological listing of past work experience, while others feel that a functional résumé detailing achievements is a more desirable approach. Some experts insist that a career objective appear at the top of the page, or it simply isn't a résumé, while others feel that employers use objectives to screen out potential employees. There is really no way to write the "perfect résumé."

A lot depends on what the potential employer is looking for, so gather as much information as you can! Talk to secretaries, other employees, friends, neighbors ... anyone who may have the "inside scoop." You are trying to gather information that will not only allow you to tailor your résumé to the needs of the company, but will also help you find out if you would enjoy working there. You are "taking the pulse" of the organization, even at this early stage, long before you ever talk to a prospective employer. Everyone takes the pulse sooner or later—most people do this *after* they are hired, which can be a little too late.

Do not make the mistake of thinking that your résumé will get you a job. If you randomly send out tons of résumés, you are not likely to hear back from many of those organizations. Your résumé will land in a big pile with a lot of other résumés and may be used as a tool to screen you *out* of an interview— in 30 seconds or less! Some authorities say that there is one job offer tendered and accepted for every 1,400 résumés that employers receive from job hunters. The only results you will guarantee yourself if you utilize your résumé in this manner are a lowered self-esteem, depression, hopelessness ... and it gets worse from there. The point to be made here is that once you put the effort into designing a résumé that best communicates your style, personality, and what you have to offer an employer, you need to utilize this tool effectively.

The most important thing to remember is that a résumé is only one aspect of the big picture of your career development. It should be a professional reflection of your job history and personal style. Used out of context (i.e., by itself instead of in conjunction with research and informational interviews) it becomes, at best, worthless. At worst, it can be a negative influence. Be aware that résumés are often used to screen out potential employees, and, generally speaking, the most endearing quality (and the one most likely to make your résumé stand out) is if *you* shine through all the proper grammar, neatness, and clarity.

Even though there is no single "recipe" for résumé writing, there *are* some general guidelines that you may find helpful:

▲ Be descriptive, yet brief. Organize your information so that it flows and is easy to read. One-page résumés are more likely to be read than longer ones.

▲ It is not necessary to include an objective. Your objective is best addressed in your cover letter. Remember, objectives can be used to screen you out, not in!

▲ Organize your information into categories, such as Career Objective (if you choose to include one), Employment History, Summary of Qualifications, Achievements, Education, and Professional Organizations/Certifications.

▲ Convey who you are and why the company should hire you. Vicki Spina, author of *Getting Hired in the '90s*, says that if you cannot list at least five solid reasons for a company to hire you, then you need to work on your self-image. (Aaargh! *Five* good reasons ... so many? Maybe I'll just stay at my current job. At least I don't have to be constantly justifying and explaining myself!) I don't know about you, but this was my initial response when I read that statement.

Spina goes on to identify some qualities companies look for in job candidates:

Able to do multiple tasks	Flexible	Open-minded
Anticipates boss's needs	Good communication skills	Positive attitude
Confident	Good follow-up skills	Problem-solver
Cooperative	Healthy	Professional
Creative	Honest	Quick learner
Dependable	Independent	Shows initiative
Detail-oriented	Intelligent	Team player
Efficient	Leadership skills	Well-rounded
		Works well under pressure

Well, I relaxed considerably after reading through this list. There probably isn't a nurse out there who doesn't have *at least* five of these qualities! Use these words and phrases on your résumé and in all of your communications to accurately portray who you are, what you have to offer, and why the organization should hire you.

▲ Use action-oriented words and phrases when describing yourself and your accomplishments. (See page 119 for some ideas.) You were certainly active when you developed these skills — let that come through in your positive, energetic description.

▲ Avoid repetition. It is boring and disorganized.

▲ Don't use the same action word or quality more than twice on your résumé.

▲ Start with your most recent position. List your job title, company name, city, and state. Always include dates, listed in months and years, so the prospective employer doesn't think you are trying to hide gaps in employment.

▲ Include part-time positions only if the work relates to the position for which you are applying. You may also want to list part-time work if you have not yet had a full-time position. If you have done extensive temporary work (also called registry, agency, rent-a-nurse, etc.), you may want to make a separate entry summarizing this experience rather than listing each company separately. For example, your entry could read:

> July 1989 to present, STAT Nursing Service, NSI, Sunrise Nursing Service. San Francisco, CA. Provided temporary staffing relief in the ICU, CCU, ER, and SDU settings. Performed duties independently while functioning as a team member in a variety of settings and hospitals.

Action words and qualities

Achieved	Designed	Maximized
Actively involved	Developed	Monitored
Adept	Devised	Motivated
Adjusted	Discovered	Negotiated
Administered	Energetic	Observed
Analyzed	Enhanced	Orchestrated
Assessed	Established	Organized
Attained	Evaluated	Originated
Authorized	Executed	Oversaw
Awarded	Facilitated	Prepared
Balanced	Formulated	Produced
Built	Generated	Promoted
Completed	Implemented	Recognized
Composed	Improved	Resolved
Contributed	Increased	Reviewed
Coordinated	Initiated	Revised
Created	Installed	Screened
Dedicated	Introduced	Solved
Delegated	Investigated	Synthesized
Delivered	Maintained	Streamlined
Demonstrated	Managed	Taught

If you are a newly graduated nurse, list part-time and summer employment related to nursing. For example:

> Summer, 1995. San Francisco County Women's Clinic. Nursing Assistant/Community Outreach Worker. Provided immunizations and community outreach services.

> September 1992 to present. St. Jude's Hospital, San Mateo, CA. Patient Care Technician. Provided patient care as directed by nursing staff to patients on a medical unit. Part-time position while in school.

New graduates may also want to include significant clinical rotations on their first résumé. For example:

Significant Clinical Rotations:

VA Medical Center, San Francisco, CA. Psychiatric-Mental Health.

University of California, San Francisco. Medical/Surgical, Pediatric Oncology.

Presbyterian Hospital, San Francisco, CA. Cardiac Step-Down, Cardiac Intensive Care.

San Francisco County Hospital. Advanced senior practicum in Medicine/HIV+ patients.

Research project completed through the Sexual Assault Resource Team (SART) at County Hospital in San Francisco, CA.

▲ Put the most important information at the top of your résumé. This means any relevant experience and/or skills should be highlighted first. The typical employer spends about 30 seconds reading your résumé before deciding whether or not to bring you in for an interview. Think about it … if you had a stack of 50 or 100 résumés to look through, what would *you* want to see first?

Some experts say that potential employers only read the top third and bottom third of the résumé! Position your information accordingly. For example, if a degree is required for a position, you may want to put your educational achievements at the top and then list your related experience and background. On the other hand, if you don't have the degree that is required for a position that you really want and know you could do well, then list your related experience (i.e., why they should hire you anyway) at the top and put your education and training last. Many people are hired for jobs that "require" a more advanced degree than they have. Ultimately, the employer wants someone who can do the job well. Convince them that you are the right person for the job.

▲ List your most recent degree first. Include the name of the college or university, your degree or major, and be sure to include any honors you may have achieved.

▲ Do not include personal information. This includes age, marital status, reasons for leaving your previous job, and salary information (unless salary history is specifically requested).

▲ If you are bilingual, be sure to list it as a skill!

▲ List professional organizations and any publications of your work only if you have the space, unless this information directly relates to the job you are seeking.

▲ "References available on request" should be the very last line on your résumé. List your references (three professional and three personal) on a separate page, matching the paper and type style used on your résumé. Have this with you to provide if and when you are asked for references.

▲ Always send a cover letter with your résumé. This letter adds more of your personality to the overall picture, explains who you are and why you are sending a résumé, and provides a personal introduction and explanation for your contact with the decision-maker rather than taking the "usual" approach through the human resources department.

▲ Do not stretch the truth. You may end up in a job that is over your head and at which you have no hope of succeeding. Also, potential employers do check references from jobs and schools.

▲ Tailor your résumé to the position you are seeking. You may want to have several different résumés, each with a different focus and content, so that you can present yourself in the best light to a variety of types of employers. If you have access to a computer, you can tailor each résumé individually

▲ ▲ ▲

Okay ... whew! Let the writing begin!

A good place to start is to organize your data. Sift through your past achievements, work history, experience, education, and all of the other information covered in Chapter 3. You will want to use this information to focus your résumé on the type of position you seek and to paint a realistic and positive picture of yourself and what you have to offer.

Review the master skills and activities list you prepared in Chapter 3. You will use these words in your résumé to start each sentence with an action word. Remember to use a variety of descriptive terms, and avoid repetition.

Now, using the sample résumés from the resource guide in the back of the book as your guide, create your own résumé or résumés. Ask your family and friends for feedback, and work on the thing until it feels *right* to you — until it feels like an accurate portrayal of you, your personality, your skills, and what you have to offer an organization. Then, stand up and do a little victory dance! You'll have completed an important step in your career development process, and you will actually have something very tangible to show for it!

Typographical tips

Use a layout that attracts attention and is easy to read. Make sure your margins are at least one inch (so there is room for notes), and put extra space between blocks of information or categories to create some "white space" — it is much easier to read.

Use an 11- or 12-point font size. If your type is too small, it is difficult to read.

Don't mix font styles. Stick to one style of type — Helvetica or Times Roman are good, standard choices. Never use scripted or other hard-to-read fonts.

Use bolding, italics, small caps, and other typographical features to highlight specifics and/or headlines.

Use bullet points only for information you want to highlight, not for each job duty.

Write in the present tense for your current position and past tense for previous ones.

Have your résumé professionally typeset (if you don't have access to a computer) and laser printed. This will give you a clean, clearly readable final product.

Choose a nice quality off-white, ivory, or gray paper. Avoid bright colors, which can be distracting and annoying! Match paper products for your cover letter, résumé, references, and envelope. Type addresses on the envelope.

Using an 8½ x 11" envelope makes a nicer presentation.

Don't use recycled paper. The ink can flake off when the paper is folded, and you can end up with entire lines of type missing.

Proofread carefully! You'd be surprised at the potential price tag of spelling or grammatical errors. It could be the factor that puts your résumé in the trash before another.

Remember to include your name, address, zip code, and phone number with area code.

INFORMATIONAL INTERVIEWS

Finally, after spending all of this time exploring past experiences and future options, developing goals and plans, learning to build alliances, and constructing a résumé that expresses the entirety of what you have to offer in the workplace, it is time to get out there and start talking to people.

Informational interviewing is a tool that, as a nurse, was an entirely foreign concept to me. It never occurred to me that *other people* might be interested in my welfare and willing to help me along the way to developing a future that would make me happy.

There may have been some casual contact with staff; for example, when I was working in the step-down-unit, you could find me cornering an ICU nurse for a few quick questions when they brought a patient down. How do you like it up there? What kind of experience do I need? Is it better than working in this place? Definitely on the right track, but worlds away from spending structured time discovering exactly what I wanted to do, carefully choosing the people to talk with, and systematically gathering information that would assist me in meeting my goals. It was, quite honestly, shocking to me that busy professionals would agree to meet with me to answer questions about my interests. During the course of planning my career change, I met with a dozen or so people for informational interviews. Only *one* person declined my request for a meeting. The rest were happy to see me, and the experience was definitely a positive one.

There is really no limit to what you can find out about potential career areas by simply going out and talking to people rather than keeping the process an intellectual one, using books and reference guides, or relying on your own understanding of various types of jobs. The informational interview provides a reality check for you. Some jobs can look and sound terrific, especially if you are very unhappy in your current position. In reality, these jobs may not be at all what you are looking for. (Remember the old saying, "The grass is always greener on the other side of the fence.") Sometimes people automatically eliminate jobs as an option just because of some preconceived notion or judgment they carry—often without even being aware of these thoughts or where they came from in the first place.

In an informational interview, you want to see *workers*—people who either do what you want to do, or something similar, in the same industry that captures your interest. Your goal here is to learn more about the profession you are interested in and/or the position you are seeking. Whether a particular organization happens to have an opening, or happens to *want* to hire you, is irrelevant at this stage. It's a nice reversal from the historical job search—*you* get to decide if you want *them*, and only then do you consider asking if they also want you.

Informational interviews can take any form, from personal meetings, to phone conversations, letters, or online with a computer. Personal contact has the extra advantage of giving you practice with interviewing skills, as well as helping to break down the fear factor that most of us carry into the interview setting. This type of interview is a chance to give and receive information. You are attempting to establish rapport with this person, to develop a professional alliance with them. This is very different than going into the situation to develop a "contact," which implies that the person is able to or will provide you with a major job lead, if not the job of your dreams. Seeking a professional alliance puts a lot less pressure on them (and you). See this person as a source of information, and make it clear that this is your agenda. Any leads that bring you the opportunity to apply or interview for a job are simply an added bonus. Don't make this your goal, or it can turn off the interviewee and cause you to miss an opportunity for a valuable alliance and exchange of information.

The informational interview provides you with the chance to have an objective party evaluate and react to your goals, approach, and presentation and give you advice about your career development plan and résumé. *Objectivity* is key here. Friends and loved ones — even peers — often listen to your goals, see you as someone they love and care about, and agree to support you in those goals no matter how outrageous they might seem. How many times has a friend or family member come to you with "*the idea*" that was going to be the answer to it all? Sometimes the response is "more power to you," even though you might be thinking "not a chance." It takes an "objective other" to look at your ideas and give you honest feedback.

For example, when I decided to make a career change years ago, I wanted to *really* go for it. Never one to do things halfway, I didn't even want to discuss possibilities that existed in the health care industry. Never mind the fact that my degree was in nursing, and it was the only field I'd worked in for the past 15 years. There were vast possibilities out there. Publishing and business had always interested me, so I wanted to switch tracks and get into one of these fields or, better yet, a job that encompassed both! So off I went with my list of people to interview. Each person was helpful, happy to talk with me, and wanted to provide me with the information I needed. But, at some point during each of these interviews, the person asked me *why I didn't want to apply all my years of experience in the health care industry.* Not one to be deterred, I reiterated my interest in business and publishing, ever seeking more referrals for other people I could talk to. Then, it was as if fate stepped in.

One of the people on my list to interview was my uncle Howard. I didn't know him that well, but I did know he'd had a long career in the business and computer industries and had worked as a successful consultant for years. Out came the goals, the plans, the hopes and dreams. Now, even though Howard has never been one to mince words, I was still stunned when he said, "Why the hell do you want to go into the cutthroat business industry when you have 15 years of experience in health care? Health care is one of the most rapidly growing industries there is!" He went on to relate the story of his experience re-entering the workforce after 20 years in the navy and what it was like to be a retired military person in the post–Vietnam era. He described how he had to avoid telling people his background because it could eliminate his chances of being hired or getting promoted. He had been forced to start over from scratch, and it wasn't easy. To do that by choice, he said, was just plain not smart.

Well, this really whipped my head around a few times. Partly due to the directness of his response and partly due to the objective clarity of his perspective on the health care industry, it finally sank in and I realized *all those people had been right*. Which didn't make me wrong, but it certainly opened my eyes to the reality of the situation. The moral of the story is, as the old saying goes, *don't throw the baby out with the bathwater*. For me to ignore four years of college and 15 years of experience in health care just because I was not satisfied with my recent jobs bordered on insane. I got back on the right track by shifting my focus to include areas within health care that would provide me with skills in business and publishing and allow me to pursue exactly what I wanted in a way that was *holistic*, that helped me to utilize my past experience, and that was realistically possible for me to achieve.

The informational interview is a meeting with another person to gather information and advice relevant to your career. Nothing more, nothing less. Do you *have* to go out and do informational interviews? Of course not. If you aren't fazed in the least by going and talking to new people, already know how to ask for the information you need, and feel excitement instead of abject terror at the thought of going on an interview, then the informational interview is not for you. It's more appropriate for those of us who are a little shy, and who don't like to go out and talk to people. Or those of us who don't have a lot of experience asking for what we need. Or those of us who are not quite certain which job we would be best suited for and happy doing, and who break out in a cold sweat at the thought of going out on interview after interview, facing rejection on jobs we we're not even sure we want. This is no joke—how many nurses do you know who feel prepared to do all the steps required to develop their career into what they always dreamed was possible?

The beauty of it is, you can take it at your own pace. If you feel shy or uncomfortable jumping into a formal informational interview, then go out and practice a bit first. Some experts suggest that you think of some topic you *love* to talk about. Whether the topic seems trivial or you feel passionate about it, it should not be connected in any way with career plans you may have. Perhaps you love cats, skiing, sewing, or children, or you feel strongly about homelessness or people with AIDS. It just needs to be something you love to talk about. The only other rule is to talk about it with someone you do not know. Check the yellow pages, ask friends and family if they know of anyone who shares your interest. If you love to sew, try the local fabric store. Cat lovers can try the pound or a local vet.

After you identify someone you think shares your interest, *go and talk to them.* Ask them for just ten minutes of their time. Then stick to your time limit, so you don't spend your time talking to someone who is anxious about how long this will take and can't focus on your conversation. Tell them that you are trying to get more comfortable with talking to people for the purpose of gathering information and that you felt the two of you might share a mutual interest ... and away you go.

The main goal here is to have fun and to have the experience of talking with "strangers" about topics of mutual interest.

You might ask how they got interested in this topic. How long have they had this interest? What do they like most and least about it? Do they know of any others who might share their enthusiasm? Is it okay to tell these people that they recommended that you contact them? Be sure to thank people for their time, and if you can recall one thing that you really valued in the exchange, be sure to tell them. For example, "I really love your suggestion that I talk to Joe at the pet shop. I had no idea that he was such a cat lover!"

It is absolutely fine to take someone along with you—a friend, associate, your mother … whoever can help you feel comfortable as you get used to talking with people about your interests. Keep going on practice interviews until you feel confident and at ease talking to people and asking questions about things you want to know. Most of all, keep doing them until you have *fun* doing them. You will know that it's time to move on when you no longer dread the idea of setting up another interview.

Be sure to send a thank-you note within 24 hours to anyone who helps you, *at any time,* during your career development journey.

Once you've become comfortable with the idea of going on an informational interview, the rest of the process is easy. There are six simple steps:

1. Compile a list of people you would like to contact;

2. Compose a letter of introduction;

3. Follow up with a phone call to set an appointment;

4. Conduct the informational interview;

5. Send a thank-you letter; and

6. Follow up with any referrals given to you during interview.

1. *Compile a list of people you would like to contact.* Examine the goals and personal action plan you developed in Chapter 6. If you are still unclear about which area of nursing to pursue, you may want to review Chapter 4 on career options to help narrow your focus. Using this information, write down at least three career options you would consider as possibilities for meeting your goals. This is only a start—you may want to refer back to your goals and plans and expand this list later. Write each of the three options on a separate page and, underneath them, write down names of people you know who work in that arena. If you don't know anyone, begin by making a list of places and/or people you could contact who might be able to recommend someone for you to interview. Keep in mind that ⅔ of all new jobs are created by small organizations—you may want to target them, rather than a Fortune 500 company. Check publications, magazines, newspaper ads, and articles— any place you might be able to identify someone who is an expert in your field of interest.

One of the most informative and enjoyable interviews I did during my search was with Karlene Kerfoot, VP of Nursing at St. Luke's Episcopal Hospital in Houston, Texas. In a very impressive interview/article in *Nursing Economic$*, she outlined her program, The Center for Innovations in Nursing, which was designed to improve quality and productivity in nursing. After I read her article and decided I'd like to speak with her, I called directory assistance to get the number for her hospital. The switchboard operator put me right through to her secretary! Asking for her time felt like a long shot, but not only did she agree to talk with me, she spent more than half an hour and offered to send articles that would help me meet my goals!

Don't be shy. The worst thing anyone can do is say no, at which point you move on to the next person. Talk to your peers, manager, or people from other departments in your company to see if they can recommend contacts. If you pursue "leads" like a private investigator, you will come up with an outstanding array of people to talk with. Start out with at least three people for each career option.

2. *Compose a letter of introduction.* Your initial contact with a potential interviewee usually takes the form of a letter—although it may be more informal, depending on who you are contacting. Let common sense be your guide, but when in doubt, send a letter. Make your letter short, clear, and to the point. Your goal here is to introduce yourself, explain why you are contacting the person, and briefly state what you hope to accomplish in a meeting with them. Advise them that you will follow up by phone. It is very important that you be *short and to the point*—long dissertations on your life path and goals will probably be set aside or trashed. Try to imagine what you would want to know if someone sent you a letter like this. *I* would want to know who this person is, how they found out about me, and what they want. Short and to the point.

An important goal in writing a letter of introduction for an informational interview is to make your expectations clear. Often people who receive this kind of letter think they are expected to get you a job or send you to someone who can. Remember the difference between a "contact" and an "alliance"? Make it clear that you are seeking information and advice, *not* expecting them to provide a contact. Bernard Haldane Associates, a nationwide marketing consultation company, suggests a statement such as: "Please understand that I do not expect you to know of or have any positions at this time. I would, however, greatly appreciate your advice and insight about _____."

For sample letters of introduction, refer to the resource guide at the end of this book. Of course, your letter should reflect *your* personality and values. Always include a copy of your résumé with the letter for them to review if they choose, and always explain *when* you will follow up with a phone call.

Wait for at least two days after they should have received your letter before you place the call.

A couple of presentation suggestions: If you have access to a computer, it is best to send a typewritten letter, which is much easier to read. Be creative, and make up letterhead—it simply needs to include your name, address, phone and fax number (if you have one available). Look at various styles of letterhead, and use a combination of what you like best in each style. It's not as hard as you might think!

Remember, choose a nice quality paper for all of your communications, including letters of introduction, cover letters, résumés, and thank-you letters. White or off-white linen paper is a good choice—any copy store or office supply store should stock them. And don't forget matching envelopes, if possible!

3. *Follow up with a phone call to set an appointment.* The main goal of the follow-up call is to set up an appointment with this person. Allow enough time for them to receive and read the letter—usually around a week from the mailing date. Don't wait too long though, or it could be misinterpreted as a loss of interest or failure to follow up. Start by identifying yourself. Then explain that you sent a letter (mention the date you sent it) and ask if they have had a chance to read it. Do not go into any long explanations of your letter, unless they ask for clarification. If they have read it, then they know why you are calling. Once you confirm that they've received the letter and know who you are, ask if it would be convenient to meet with you. Suggest a date and time, or at least say "next week." Don't just say "any time is fine with me." Of course, you want to be flexible, and accommodate their schedule.

If you are uncomfortable at first, write out a script and keep it in front of you while you are on the phone. If *they* seem uncomfortable or uncertain, it may be useful to remind them that you are only seeking information about the work they do and that you don't expect them to know of any positions at this time. If it is difficult to nail down an appointment time, then be as flexible as possible and schedule *something*, even if it is a couple of weeks away. For appointments more than a couple of weeks in the future, you may want to send a "reminder letter" mentioning your conversation and scheduled meeting time. It is always worthwhile to make a phone call the day before to confirm the appointment. It's a hassle and somewhat embarrassing to show up at someone's office when the person has totally forgotten an appointment with you, or the secretary forgot to cancel...

If the person has not received your letter when you first call, offer to call back in a couple of days. If there is still no letter, then confirm the address, send another copy, and follow through with a phone call as above.

It is always best to meet with someone in person, but occasionally you might want to talk with someone who lives a long distance away. Unless you are independently wealthy and can fly around as much as you want, you may choose to do some interviews by phone. Although there are certain limitations in not meeting face to face, some of the best interviews I ever did were by phone. Common sense, practicality, and flexibility are your best guides, as they are throughout this entire process.

4. *Conduct the informational interview.* Although there is really no recipe for how an informational interview "should" be carried out, there are some guidelines you may find useful.

▲ Arrive 10 to 15 minutes early. For heaven's sake, *do not* be late!

▲ Your first job is to establish some type of rapport with this person. Look around the office for pictures that may give you an idea of a shared interest, or even talk about the weather, if you must. It just helps to break the ice.

▲ After a few minutes of chatting, bring the meeting into focus. You can end up wasting a lot of time if the meeting stays too chatty or informal. You may want to say something like: "Since we only have a limited amount of time together, I'll get right to the point."

▲ Start with a brief introduction. Thank your interviewee for taking the time to see you, and reassure them that you do not expect that they will have or know of a job for you at this time. State the purpose of your visit. For example: "I am currently exploring career options in which I can apply my skills in leadership and analysis. In a recent conversation with Brad Jones, he recommended that I contact you as a source of information and advice on how my clinical application of these skills could be transferred into the QA/UR arena."

▲ Be prepared to tell this person about you and your skills. Use your résumé as a guide, and be sure the interviewee understands what you say. You might even ask at the end, "Do you believe my skills and background are consistent with my objective?"

▲ Once you are certain that the interviewee understands your objective for the meeting, then proceed with your prepared questions.

▲ If you want to use notes for your questions or jot down ideas during the interview, it is always polite to ask the person if it is okay for you to take notes.

▲ Be sure to give the person enough time to think and respond.

▲ Listen. Carefully and actively listen.

▲ Pay attention to body language. You can gather lots of information from these unspoken cues as to how the person feels about the job and the organization.

▲ Don't be afraid to ask someone to clarify or expand on a particularly interesting point.

▲ Wait until the end of the interview to ask for referrals.

▲ Always ask if it is okay for you to use their name when contacting the referrals they may offer.

▲ Thank the interviewee for their time.

▲ You may want to ask if it would be okay for you to stay in touch and keep them apprised of your progress. This can leave the door open for future contact if they have shown a real interest in you.

▲ Send a thank-you note within 24 hours.

If you keep in mind the purpose of the informational interview (meeting with someone to gather information and advice relevant to your career), it can take the edge off the "interview stigma" so many of us carry. You may want to call it something else, such as a career advice session. No matter what you call it, the clearer you are about what you are doing and what you hope to accomplish, the more enjoyable the interview will be for you.

The key to walking into an informational interview with enough clarity to enjoy the process is to *prepare*. Think very carefully about your purpose for going to see each person. Be clear about what you hope to accomplish in the meeting and what information you want to gather. Remember, since *you* have requested the meeting, it is *your* responsibility to be prepared and to run the interview. This preparation needs to be done before you are face-to-face with your interviewee.

It is important to understand what you want to accomplish during your interviewing process. There are three main objectives when you go on an informational interview:

1. You want the person being interviewed to *help you understand which types of careers can best utilize your training, skills, experiences, and interests.*

2. If the person works in an area that interests you, you may also want them to *give you some idea of what that type of work is like.*

3. If the contact does not work in your area of interest and doesn't know what it is like, then you want to *ask for the names of people who do work in that arena, and go and talk to them.*

Let's get more specific about how to effectively prepare for the informational interview. Using the above objectives, each step can be broken down and clarified. Our goal here is to gather the appropriate information in each of these three areas to ensure a successful interview.

▲ You want to gain an understanding of which careers could best utilize your training, skills, experiences, and interests. In order for the people you are interviewing to provide you with this information and advice, they are going to need to know about you. This means you must be able to clearly and succinctly present your training, skills, experience, and interests to them.

You will already have supplied them with some information—the moment they received your letter and résumé, you were communicating loudly and clearly. These documents are tools that assist you in communicating to the interviewee. Be sure they reflect honestly who you are, what you have done, and where you want to go. Always bring a copy of your résumé to the meeting. (I know ... you sent one with the letter. But what if they do not have it handy, or they lost it?) You can use the résumé as a guide while you give them a brief introduction and summary of your training, skills, experience, and interests.

Discuss the skills you most enjoy using and wish to develop, as well as your current objectives. In the business world, this is often called the "two-minute drill." This phrase made me want to panic, but it does aptly capture the importance of getting this information out in a clear manner—short and to the point. Work on this introduction before you go to the interview. Write it out. Time yourself. Ask your family and/or pets to listen to you as you practice. You may want to make a recording and listen to yourself.

Personally, I never had a problem getting this information out in two minutes or less. My tendency was to get sort of flustered and embarrassed at talking about myself and skip over a lot of details with a sort of "well, you know..." kind of attitude. Well, they *don't* know, and after a couple of interviews, it was very clear that these people wanted to help me, wanted to know about me, and were interested in what I had to tell them. After this realization, it became more embarrassing to leave out the details and not give them a clear picture of who I was and what I had to offer than it was to just give them the whole "drill." Think of it as a change of shift report—you need to provide them with all the vital statistics so that they can provide appropriate care. It's really not as hard as it seems.

After you finish your two-minute introduction, a good question to ask is: "Based on what I have told you, how do you see someone with my training, skills, experience, and interests making the transition from _____ to _____ ?" This is a broad question which gives you an opportunity to evaluate how your information was received, if it was understood, and where you may need to clarify. Getting feedback on how they see you fitting into their industry is a good first step.

▲ You want to find out what that type of work is like. In order to gather this information, you need to come prepared with some good questions. Remember, you are the one who is responsible for guiding the interview. So have the questions written out, and keep them handy for easy reference. But don't go overboard and become obsessed with the list! It is important to let the topic roam a bit. Just because you have the questions written down in a certain order doesn't mean that they have to be answered in a systematic way. Be familiar enough with your questions to recognize the answers when they come in a conversational manner. Most people enjoy talking about their jobs and their careers. If you allow the conversation to follow its own natural course, you'll still get the answers you are after and may gain even more honest or candid information along the way. However, you may need to use the questions to bring your goal back into focus if things get *too* casual.

Questions should be open-ended, not closed. For example, "Do you like your work?" could be answered with a simple yes or no, whereas, "What do you like most and least about your work?" encourages an open discussion about likes and dislikes.

▲ You want to gather names of others who may be helpful sources of information. The end of the interview, after you have established a rapport with the interviewee and been engaged in an exchange of information for a period of time, is the best time to ask for one or two people you might talk to for additional advice. Always ask for referrals before you leave, and be sure all interviewees understand that you will not be asking these people for a job, but will be seeking information just as you did from them. You may want to ask for people who are versed in your specific area of interest. If your interviewee cannot think of someone right away, offer to give them some time to think and call back in a few days. Set a date to make this telephone contact before you leave the interview. Then be sure to follow through.

Don't be shy about asking for more than one name, but remember that *quality* is far more important than quantity when it comes to referrals. You can gather more important information in one good interview than in ten mediocre ones.

5. *Send a thank-you letter.* No matter how the interview went, or how you may feel about how it went, *everyone* gets a thank-you letter. This is a powerful tool that provides a positive feeling of closure to the exchange. Your thank-you should reflect your own personal style. Some people prefer to send a handwritten note, while others feel it is more professional to send a typed letter. The person you interviewed has to be taken into account, as well. If someone has a more formal demeanor, a letter would probably be the appropriate approach. If the person is a friend of a friend and the interview was very casual, then it may make better sense to send a note. The most important thing is that you send it, and send it promptly! Get it in the mail the next day, at the latest. Not only is this proper etiquette, it is just plain polite. This person took the time to show an interest in you and your career. They deserve your thanks! Be honest in your letter, and always try to reference something of value that the person said or advised. If you discussed keeping in touch after the interview, you may want to mention this again now.

For a sample thank-you letter, refer to the resource guide at the end of this book.

6. *Follow up on any referrals you were given.* You never know where the key piece of information will come from, or who will provide the exact link-up your brain needs to become clear about how you wish to proceed. The person who gave you the referral may mention it to that person, and then you will look like a flake if you don't follow through. This happened to me recently. A woman approached me and asked for an informational interview to help her understand the field of medical sales. We set a meeting, had a terrific exchange, and I provided her with the names of two sales contacts. Unbeknownst to her,

I also left a message for them to let them know I'd referred her so they would be expecting her call. Well, there never *was* a call. Made her look bad. Could've made me look bad. Don't do this. If you ask for names, do your follow-up.

Another tip: When I was deep in the process of interviewing, it sometimes felt difficult to keep track of who I talked to, when, what they said, the referrals they gave me … and, oh yeah, did I ever send that thank-you note? Good record keeping decreases the chance that you will leave someone wondering what happened to you, why you didn't call as agreed, why you didn't send a thank-you, or why you never contacted the referrals they gave you. All of this reflects poorly on you. It can be easy to keep track of all this information if you just create some simple forms that you can fill out as you go. You need only the basics, such as their name, who referred you to them, phone number, address, date of your initial contact letter, date of telephone contact, date of interview, names of referrals obtained, date your thank-you was sent, and dates for follow-up calls and/or interviews. You may also want to add small sections for other information, such as a description of the interview, any pertinent information or advice that was obtained, and any planned follow-through.

COVER LETTERS

The purpose of the informational interview is to gather information about your job options, which employers to contact, starting salary figures, and the names and titles of contacts. As you compile this information, you will start to sense openings, or leads, that you may wish to pursue. Maybe several of your interviewees raved about a certain company and the opportunities they'd heard of there. Or perhaps someone said, "Contact Jane Smith at Quality Review, Inc. I know she is looking for someone, and I think she'd like you." The time will come for you to take the next step: secure a job interview.

Before you do anything else, however, take the time to do a quick brush-up on your résumé. Use the feedback you've gotten from your informational interviews, your friends, peers, and family to guide any changes you may want to make. Then, it is time to compose your cover letter.

Your cover letter is as important as your résumé! It is your introduction, your first impression. This little one-page letter should reflect your unique personal skills and abilities. No, this is not impossible! Although many people are intimidated by the prospect of writing a cover letter, it becomes easier if you break it down into its three main components:

1. *What you want.* This includes the type of opportunity and/or position you are seeking and why you are looking for a job.

2. *What you have to offer.* Emphasize what you can bring to the job and any related experiences or specific achievements that demonstrate your capacity for success. Point out what would make you uniquely valuable to them and how you could meet their needs.

3. *Your availability for an interview.* Close your letter by stating that you will be calling to discuss job opportunities and your availability for an interview. Be specific—for example, "I will call you next week." The only time you would not want to include this statement is if the person specifically stated they would contact you. In this case, you could close with something like: "I look forward to hearing from you and learning more about job opportunities at _____ ."

In addition to the above components, the following guidelines may help demystify the cover letter and its appropriate use:

▲ Always send a cover letter with your résumé. It is your introduction in absentia.

▲ Submit a résumé with a cover letter even if you have been asked to fill out an application that contains all the information. This demonstrates initiative, professionalism, organizational skills, and courtesy.

▲ Each cover letter needs to be individually created and geared specifically to the position for which you are applying.

▲ Always send your letter and résumé to the individual who is most likely to be the decision-maker about who gets the job. This may require some detective work. A few phone calls will often lead you to the name of this person, or you may receive the name from a friend, family member, or in an informational interview. If you send your résumé to the personnel or human relations department, you may as well kiss it good-bye. These departments frequently use résumés to screen *out* applicants.

▲ If you are sending an unsolicited résumé or heard about an opening from someone else, simply include an explanation of how you heard about the company.

▲ Make sure your stationery matches or complements your résumé.

▲ Start your letter with a complimentary statement or information you've discovered about the company.

▲ Incorporate your unique skills and abilities in this letter. Use action words to interject a positive, enthusiastic tone.

▲ Be sure you spell names correctly, list their most recent job title, and have an accurate address. Mistakes in these areas can be embarrassing and/or cause delays. Call to verify!

▲ Keep it short—one page is best.

▲ Make the letter a personable and accurate presentation of yourself.

Sample cover letters can be found in the resource guide at the end of this book.

The follow-up call to sending your cover letter and résumé is similar to the calls you made for informational interviews. Basically, the same rules apply, so review the "follow-up calls to informational interviews" section on page 132. The main goal is to set up an appointment to meet this person face-to-face.

JOB INTERVIEWS

So, now all your hard work has paid off—you've been invited to come in for a job interview. Dry off your sweaty palms ... you are prepared! Right? Because, surely you know at this point that *preparation is essential.* By now you understand that the goal of the interviewer may very well be to screen you in *or out* of the position. But if you've done your homework, you will be prepared to overcome any initial trepidation and use the interview process as a tool to help you find the "right match." It's an exchange of information and ideas. (Okay, so it's also the arena in which you are sized up by the potential employer—remember, you are sizing them up, too!)

Your preparation actually began a long time ago. The informational interview played a key role in your preparation by helping you get used to talking with people about mutual interests and feel less nervous about the interviewing process. Now it is time to prepare in a way that is very specific to this organization and this interviewer.

First, find out as much about the organization as you can. Who are the key people? What is their primary product or service? Company size, sales, number of employees, locations, industry growth rate, how the company is perceived by its clients, suppliers, competition ... all of this information helps you begin to put together a view of the organization. Talk to current and former employees (you may find an informational interview with some of them to be beneficial), study annual reports, journal and newspaper articles, and talk to your friends and business associates. Then, study the information and start preparing intelligent questions to ask during the interview.

It is also a good idea to find out all you can about the responsibilities of the position, what the interviewer's long-range goals are, and how they plan to reach them. Keep in mind, the interview process is a *two-way street.* Use it to gather more information about the organization and your potential boss to help you decide if you really want to work there.

Once you have some information about the company and the position, spend some time thinking about what you are willing to accept in terms of hours, working conditions, salary, and other terms of employment. No decisions need to be made at this point, but it's helpful to have some idea of your bottom line. You may want to divide your hourly or monthly income by the number of hours you *really* work—commute time and preparation time included—to get a clearer picture of what you earn. I'm here to tell you, this can be an enlightening exercise!

Next, rather than worrying about what kind of questions you will be asked, *anticipate* those questions and practice your answers. Think about what the employer would be trying to find out about you. There are numerous books available on "power interviewing." Many are excellent references and list page after page of potential interview questions that you can and should anticipate. Usually, they all boil down to five simple questions:

1. "Why did you pick *our* organization instead of seeking a job somewhere else?"

2. "What are your skills and achievements, and do they match our needs?"

3. "What kind of person are you?"

4. "What sets you apart from all the other people who can do the same thing?"

5. "Can we afford you?"

Even if none of the above questions are ever actually spoken out loud, they can be found under the surface of nearly every question asked. So, this is good news! Only five questions to prepare for! But ... you'd best *know* those five answers! This should be easy if you've completed the exercises in Chapter 3. If you haven't ... well, it's not too late!

Be aware that many interviewers will throw out some difficult questions, often as a means of "testing" you. This is not necessarily done just to watch you squirm. Difficult or sensitive questions are used in an attempt to gather information and assess your compatibility, attitude, and problem-solving style ... all of which tell the interviewer how you might fit into the organization, what type of leadership style you have, and how well you function under pressure. The interviewer's emotional response can play an important role in their decision to offer you a position or not. It is said that 90% of the hiring decision is based on your personality and how well the interviewer likes you. If you have an understanding of the purpose of their questions, chances are you will be better able to keep your wits about you and provide the information they are *really* seeking rather than getting nervous or testy in response. Just be yourself, tell the truth, and bring along your sense of humor!

There is very little that will *not* be seen by the interviewer. Things like your posture, body language, hair style, manner of dress, smell (i.e., heavy perfume, cologne, smoke, breath, body odor), fingernails (clipped, clean?), whether you interrupt, are hesitant or self-assured, prepared or unprepared, enthusiastic or unenthusiastic, the sound of your voice ... all will be noticed by the interviewer. (Incidentally, non-smokers win out 94% of the time, according to a study done at Seattle University.) If you meet over lunch, it will be noticed if you order a drink or not (don't), and whether you show courtesy to the server (do). It is *always* in your best interest to be courteous and friendly with the secretary and other people in the office of the interviewer. Word really does get around, and pretty much everything will become a piece of the puzzle this person is trying to put together that answers the question, "What kind of a person is this?"

There are some traits that are a definite turn-off for most employers: lack of enthusiasm, arrogance, complaining, blaming things on others, griping about your old boss (a definite no-no … remember Mom's rule: "If you can't say anything nice, *don't say anything at all!*"), instability, inappropriateness, dishonesty, interrupting and tardiness. Once again, common sense prevails. Be yourself. If you are really *are* someone who is dishonest, rude, and unstable, then it is probably best to get those cards out on the table. But don't, out of nervousness, give someone the wrong impression about you. First impressions really do make a difference. If you are courteous toward every person you come into contact with, including the interviewer, and don't "bad mouth" your previous employers, you will likely be remembered for your graciousness. Also, it may be worth your time to read a book or some articles on how to project a positive, professional image.

Now, just as the hundreds of interview questions to anticipate were distilled into five basic ones, so can the questions that *you* must find the answers for during the interview be distilled. They are:

1.   What does this job require?

2.   Are my skills a "good match" for this job?

3. Are these the kind of people I enjoy working with?

4. What sets me apart from all the others who can also do this job, and how can I convey this to you?

5. Can I persuade you to hire me and pay me the salary I want?

Keep these questions running in your head like a feedback-loop tape throughout your interview. Five questions for them, five questions for you. Simple, right? See how balanced that is? It is no accident, believe me. A researcher at the Massachusetts Institute of Technology found that, generally speaking, the people who get hired are those who mix speaking and listening 50-50 during the interview. Makes sense, when you think about it. If you talk too much about yourself, you may come off as egotistical and arrogant — not likely to be concerned about the needs of the organization. In fact, most studies indicate that you should speak for no longer than two minutes at a time if you want to make the best impression. If you talk too little, they may get the impression that you are not a strong, capable, independent worker, or that you are trying to hide something. There can be a real sense of easy flow to an interview that has this equal give-and-take quality, with short and clear answers and comments given by both parties. This is the flow to strive for to ensure a positive, effective exchange of information.

When the interview is over, you can save yourself a lot of unnecessary worry and wondering if you simply ask when you can expect to hear from the interviewer, and if you may contact them if for some reason they haven't gotten back to you by that time. Keep your word, and don't call before the time you agree upon. If you do end up contacting the interviewer, and things are still up in the air, then ask the same questions again.

Job interview tips

Wear simple, professional clothing. Be careful not to wear too much perfume or cologne!

Arrive 10 to 15 minutes early. Be sure you know how to get there! If you can't get there on time, call and let the interviewer know your expected arrival time.

Look purposeful while waiting . . . review your résumé, or read a magazine. You will probably be making your first impression before you even realize anyone has seen you.

Be ready with a handshake (this is true for women as well as men) but wait until the interviewer extends a hand first. Shaking hands is not "standard practice" in nursing the way it is in business. Avoid an awkward moment by being prepared to offer a firm handshake when requested. It is not unusual for interviewers to eliminate candidates because of a weak or clammy handshake.

Be prepared. Carry several copies of your résumé with you, as well as your list of references to be provided on request. Take extra money in case of unforeseen expenses.

Be aware of your nonverbal communication. Maintain eye contact.

Be concise, yet informative. Remember to keep your responses under two minutes in length.

Don't bring a friend or relative along with you.

Don't smoke, chew gum, or interrupt the interviewer.

Never make negative comments about a previous company or boss.

Be honest, and don't feel as if you have to agree with everything the interviewer says.

Job interview tips (continued)

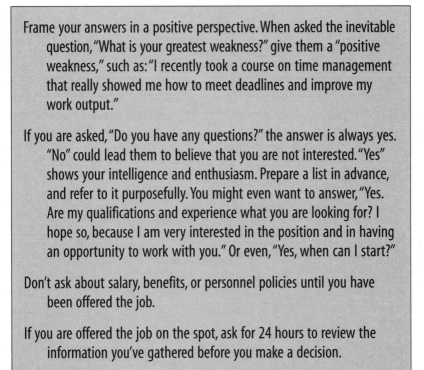

Frame your answers in a positive perspective. When asked the inevitable question, "What is your greatest weakness?" give them a "positive weakness," such as: "I recently took a course on time management that really showed me how to meet deadlines and improve my work output."

If you are asked, "Do you have any questions?" the answer is always yes. "No" could lead them to believe that you are not interested. "Yes" shows your intelligence and enthusiasm. Prepare a list in advance, and refer to it purposefully. You might even want to answer, "Yes. Are my qualifications and experience what you are looking for? I hope so, because I am very interested in the position and in having an opportunity to work with you." Or even, "Yes, when can I start?"

Don't ask about salary, benefits, or personnel policies until you have been offered the job.

If you are offered the job on the spot, ask for 24 hours to review the information you've gathered before you make a decision.

Arrange for follow-up.

THANK-YOU LETTERS

As with informational interviews, *every* person you talk to should receive a note of thanks. This is best done immediately after the interview; it should be *in the mail* by the next morning, at the latest. Write a letter that lets the interviewer know you listened carefully. Somehow let them know that you are aware of their needs and/or problems, and that you are prepared to offer a significant contribution to the organization. Add something specific about the way you were treated or something they said. Your letter should be enthusiastic, but be sure the tone is consistent with the tone of your behavior during the interview (have you ever noticed how some people communicate in an entirely different manner when they are writing than when they are speaking?). Use this opportunity to mention anything you may have forgotten while you were there, emphasize points you want the interviewer to remember about you, and reiterate your interest in speaking with them again.

There are sample thank-you letters in the resource guide at the end of this book.

A FEW WORDS ABOUT MONEY

Salary etiquette seems to be one of those areas where nursing separates from business in a big way. In the business world, there are some very simple rules. No one can tell me exactly where they come from, but they are, across the board, accepted as rules:

- ▲ *Never* discuss salary until you have been offered a position.

- ▲ *Never* be the first one to mention a salary figure.

- ▲ *Do your homework* on how much you need to earn.

- ▲ *Determine,* to the best of your ability, if the salary being offered has any room for negotiation.

- ▲ *Always* do your research, and know the standard salary range for the position you're interviewing for.

- ▲ Oh yeah, and *never* let them see you sweat.

In the world of nursing, however, many interviewers want to know your previous salary right up front. Sometimes, it's the first question they'll ask. In addition, they don't necessarily respond well to someone who avoids giving a direct answer. Many nursing positions are salaried, with a fixed hourly or monthly wage. But don't be fooled. Most "fixed" salaries exist within a range, and there is usually at least *some* wiggle room. It can be a delicate dance to honor the culture of the interviewer while still keeping the door open for the highest salary you can negotiate.

Even though the rules may be somewhat different in nursing, it is still of value to know the tricks of the trade for salary negotiation. Pulled into the appropriate perspective, these tools can be of great help in allowing you to feel more like a participant, rather than a subject, in the process of negotiation. So, always do your very best to remember these rules and, whenever possible:

▲ *Never discuss salary until you have been offered a position.* If salary is, indeed, one of the first questions asked, you can politely ask that they first help you understand what the job involves. Then try to keep the discussion focused on the job rather than the pay. If the interviewer continues to press for an answer, you may want to respond with some kind of salary range. If the person insists on a specific figure, you're pretty much out of luck. Salary negotiation is not likely to happen.

Many employers are making salary one of their key criteria for hiring in today's tight job market, and if you try to avoid answering, you lose. If you give the wrong answer, you lose. When you run into someone like this, and you want the job badly enough, you really have no choice but to ask what is offered and take it from there.

▲ *Never be the first one to mention a salary figure.* There are probably lots of reasons for this rule, but the bottom line is this: *Whoever mentions a salary figure first, is generally in a weaker position in the end.* Your interviewer may or may not know this. But experienced interviewers probably do—that's why they will *always* toss the ball to you by asking you what kind of salary you are looking for. So, now that you, too, know this general rule, you will *always* be prepared to respond by saying something like: "You must have some figure in mind, and I'd be interested in knowing what that is."

▲ *Do your homework on how much you need to earn.* If and when that time comes, it is not possible to negotiate unless you know your own salary requirements. This means you must be clear about the highest salary you would hope to earn and the absolute lowest amount you could afford to accept. It is very important to know your own bottom line.

If there is no way they can pay you what you absolutely need to earn, then you are better off looking elsewhere. (Have you ever been happy with a job that didn't pay you enough money to be comfortable?) On the other hand, you must factor in a potential decrease in income when you make a transition from one type of nursing to another. For example, it is often necessary to take a cut in pay when you move from the hospital setting to home health or quality assurance. Consider all aspects of reward in the process of deciding your bottom line (hours, work environment, growth and promotion potential, happiness, etc.). The clearer you are about your bottom line, the easier it will be to negotiate a salary and make a decision about whether this is the "right" job.

▲ *Determine, to the best of your ability, if the salary being offered has any room for negotiation.* Salary negotiation has definitely never been an easy task. It is even more challenging these days because of the widespread cost-cutting we have all become painfully familiar with in recent years. Cost is sometimes *the* deciding factor when an employer is faced with more than one attractive candidate. It is, however, not impossible to negotiate a better salary. The best way to get an idea of how much wiggle room exists in an offer is to carefully do your research on salary ranges.

▲ *Always do your research, and know the standard salary range for the position you're interviewing for.* The standard salary range for the position you are interviewing for is an important piece of information to have when you walk into an interview. Hopefully, this was included in the list of questions you took to your informational interviews, and you already have a good idea of the range to expect. If this is not the case, get out and *talk to people.* Ask someone who is in the same job at a different organization, or someone at the university or other institution where people are trained for this type of work. Check with college placement offices. Read the want ads. And, as always, talk to friends, family, and peers (as appropriate). You never know who might know what. As a last resort, there are books at the library that list occupations and salary ranges—ask your local librarian.

When the time comes and the employer tells you the figure the organization has in mind, you want to be prepared enough to respond by saying something like: "I understand the financial constraints that all health care organizations are facing these days, but I believe that my background, skills, and productivity are such that they *justify* a salary in the range of _____ ," and then mention a figure near the top of their range. Be prepared to explain *how* you could make them money or save them money. And remember to pay attention to "fringe benefits." Health and life insurance, vacation, holidays, and retirement programs can add 25 to 30% to your salary and often can be negotiated when the salary cannot. Be sure to ask when you could expect to be in line for a raise, if you perform to their satisfaction. Take time, if you need it, to add all of this up, and weigh the pros and cons carefully before accepting a position. Once all is said and done, hands are shaken, and everyone is happy, ask for a summary of your agreement in writing (in an "offer letter"). The road to hell is paved with oral promises that were unwritten, and—later—unfulfilled. If you don't receive an offer letter, you can send an "acceptance letter" which details your understanding of the oral agreement. An example of an acceptance letter can be found in the resource guide at the end of this book.

JOB OFFERS

Finally, and perhaps most importantly, *don't accept a job unless it is just what you want.* It would be a shame to waste all this hard work, wouldn't it? Plus, chances are pretty good that you'd end up right back in the same ol' kettle of soup and, in a couple of years, be doing this all over again. Hold out for what you really want, because *it is out there*, and *you can find it.* You would be cheating yourself by lapsing into the gotta-getta-job-and-gotta-get-it-now mentality at this point.

Teachers and gurus (and business consultants!) have long described the process of "listening" to your body to know the truth. They say that your body never lies about what it's feeling. Using this time-honored technique can be helpful. For example, when you visualize yourself in this new position, do you feel your heart lift? Do you feel excited, happy, or even thrilled? Then go for it! If, however, you feel uneasy in the pit in your stomach or a sense of sadness in your heart, you may want to think long and hard before you accept the position. Pity the person who accepts a mediocre job, because they may come across the job of their dreams the next day. Or, worse yet, they might *not* make the contact that *was there* because they took themselves out of the running too soon. Do not let this happen to you!

Evaluation

CHAPTER 8

Achieving Success!

Ahh, success at last! High atop a mountain, savoring the overall view, the "big picture" of your life, your dreams, your future... But wait! Is this *real?* Is this your authentic self, or is it an image you've created to honor the sense of completion you feel after such focused work on goals? If you truly want to be your own master, mentor, and/or guru, then understanding the nature of success and what it means to you is a step you simply cannot skip.

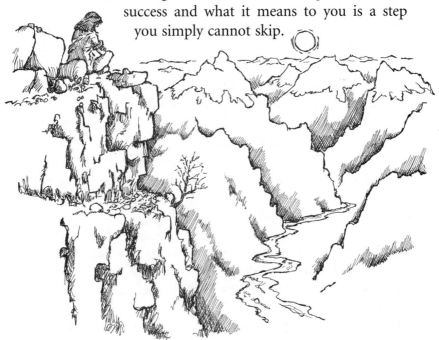

WHAT DOES SUCCESS MEAN TO YOU?

The *American Heritage College Dictionary* defines success as "the achievement of something desired, planned, or attempted." Sounds pretty straightforward, right? But then there is a second definition: "the gaining of fame or prosperity, and the extent of such gain." An entirely different story! It is fascinating to me that we live in a culture that has become so tied to the importance of material gain that it is literally linked, by definition, to the achievement of our goals. To some degree, even our deepest, most personal goals and achievements end up getting measured by the "material" ruler and dragged into the material domain because of this link.

The meaning of success is actually very personal and highly individual. Ideally, success should be defined in our own terms. When you think about it, doesn't it make sense that only *you* can know what is "successful" for you? Many native American cultures believe that each individual is "original medicine," and that there is no one like you anywhere else on the planet. Therefore, it is extremely important that we as individuals bring our life dreams and purposes to fruition. *Not* doing so prevents fulfillment from coming into our personal and professional lives. Since each person is original medicine, these cultures see no need for comparison or competition. The challenge is to bring our unique talents, gifts, and resources fully into the world. The individual contributions of many people make up the whole. When we try to follow someone else's "recipe for success," we take our very important personal contribution out of the big picture.

Our values play a powerful role in determining what we see as successful. Small wonder, then, that most people enter into slippery terrain when they start pondering success and what it means for them. Like comparing apples to oranges, comparing what success means to you with *any* other definition of success is a losing proposition. It depends on what you *value*—and how well you *understand* these values.

If we do not have a clear understanding of our values as determiners of our success, we often get locked into *society's* definition of success. In that cruel, competitive arena, our inner critic may take over, demanding that we achieve loftier and loftier goals and dismissing our past achievements as meaningless. We compare ourselves to our mother, father, brother, sister, Mother Teresa, Ghandi, and even God rather than simply focusing on ourselves. And, this is where the entire process you've just gone through can backfire if it's not kept in proper perspective.

Now, don't get me wrong here. I *personally* know the value of walking through the processes and exercises in Chapter 3. At no other time in my life had I examined my career with such scrutiny. I came out of that process with a much deeper understanding of who I am, where I've been, and where I want to go. I also had to face the pitfall, the mental mind-trap, that is inherent in the process of setting goals.

That pitfall is living life with a Goal. Note the capital G here. It is capitalized to signify the Grand Goal, the Goal like no other: my Destiny, Life's Work, and the Object of all my time, energy and devotion. Turning goals into Grand Goals is the mental mind-trap that is the downfall of many a goal-setter and begins the process of getting further and further away from your authentic self—certainly not the objective of all this hard work!

In his book, *Living Without a Goal,* James Ogilvy describes this pitfall: "A life with a single Grand Goal robs you of your freedom, because a life devoted to a single Goal demands that every action serve that single end." Grand Goals can be like huge sucking vortexes that consume all of our time and energy, becoming the object of all our attention and focus. A Grand Goal can become an obsession that causes us to adopt a sort of tunnel vision—as if anything that doesn't directly pertain to the Goal does not exist. Pursuit of a Grand Goal can cause us to miss a lot of life, to negotiate tradeoffs we often aren't even aware of. It can be a painful realization to turn around one day and realize all that you overlooked in pursuit of your Grand Goal. Many, many people are walking away from high-powered corporate jobs for just this reason—they've realized that they are missing out on *life* to pursue their Goals.

This might sound a bit extreme to you, but think about it. How many people do you know who hit the famous "midlife crisis" stage of development and came face-to-face with the fear that they had somehow missed their destiny? Do you know anyone who did a radical refocus at that time, becoming obsessed with achieving certain Goals, at all costs, before it was too late? Of course, midlife is not the only time this can happen. Anyone can fall into the mental trap of believing that the value of life depends upon the achievement of the Grand Goal, the Destiny, the Life Purpose. It is a seductive trap. Ogilvy says:

> *"Goals are so good for giving direction to a life. They are such good organizers of actions. Single-mindedness, for what it's worth, becomes possible. With a single Goal shining like a beacon on the horizon, navigation is easy: just aim for that point source of light and full steam ahead."*

But what if you have your pedal to the metal and you encounter one of those pesky changes that seem to happen about every 60 seconds these days? Can you just blast through when your Grand Goal is in direct conflict with the most recent reorganization? Not likely.

The problem here is not goals in general. Developing goals is an important part of guiding yourself through life. The exer-

160

cises you did earlier in this book were so much more than just setting goals and getting a plan together. They were tools to aid you in the process of claiming *you*. Of valuing yourself enough to pursue your dreams. Of increasing your sense of self, enlarging your world, and empowering yourself. Of building the future, the career, that you've always wanted. The problem arises when goals become Goals. *Grand* Goals. Larger than life. Determiners of inner value and self-esteem. Measurers of success, fame, and prosperity.

Grand Goals pull us out of the *here and now* and move us into the future, as if the future had the same solidity or determinacy as the past. As if we could actually *live* in the future, rather than *move toward* the future. When you live in the future, you miss the now—and the here and now is the alive, vibrant moment that, breath by breath, takes you into your future. The now is what allows you to direct your actions to *create* the future you desire. So, don't throw away your list of goals yet! Your goals are tools that you can use to direct your actions *today* to move you toward the future you desire *tomorrow*.

When you go to the corner store to get a newspaper, you have a goal. When you plan and prepare a meal, you have a goal. Goals play an enormous role in our daily lives. They are the determiners of our choices and actions. But, if the corner store is out of newspapers, does it throw you into a state of existential angst because you haven't achieved your Goal? If you burn the roast you were preparing for dinner, does that somehow imply failure as a human being? Of course not—these goals are held in the proper perspective. They are not linked as strongly to *success* as our career goals.

Perspective on career goals becomes extremely important in order to avoid the pitfalls and mind-traps associated with success. Ogilvy summarizes it well:

"Living without a Goal requires neither the optimism of a secure future nor the pessimism of hopelessness. Goal-lessness is neither a matter of counting on the promise of better days to come nor abandoning hopes of same. Things might get better; they might not. Who can tell? Living without a Grand Goal while orchestrating many goals offers opportunities for free choice, design, intelligence, and play."

Take a few moments now and contemplate your perceptions of success. How much of a role have Grand Goals played in your life, your decisions, and your relationships? You may want to return to Chapters 3 and 6 to review the results of the exercises you did there. First, look at your values clarification from Chapter 3. Can you find any pitfalls or mind-traps among them? Or are they in alignment with your big-picture view of your life? Carefully examine the goals you developed in Chapter 6. Note any new insights you may have gained since you initially wrote them. You may find it useful and thought-provoking to return to your stated values and goals periodically; it is amazing how much your perspective shifts with life experience! The values are generally pretty constant, although you will probably be viewing them through different eyes.

HOW WILL YOU KNOW WHEN YOU GET THERE?

Actually, this is a trick question. Unfortunately, it is a question that we not only ask ourselves, but will be asked by every Tom, Dick, and Harry who feels like commenting on our lives. It is a sad fact that our society is solidly achievement-based. And we're not talking about intangible achievements here! People want something they can at least *see*, and preferably something they can hold in their hand! Just try responding to someone's question about your progress on a particular project by saying that you have taken great strides toward feeling more confident that you can do the job well. Can you imagine the response? And yet, developing the self-confidence required for *any* job is truly an important first step to be mastered!

It is also a sad fact that our society has a somewhat distorted view of success and has different rules for different people. Baseball players are considered great hitters if they make just 30% of their hits. Studies have shown that the average person goes through seven to eight attempts before achieving success in their chosen endeavors. Seven to eight! Do you know of any nurses who allow themselves that many "failures"? Many well-respected, highly "successful" businessmen in this country (like Donald Trump, for example) have probably *lost* as much or more money than they have *earned*—maybe even filed bank-ruptcy—yet they are considered to be tycoons in the business world.

Most "ordinary" people do not see success from this angle. We're afraid to take the risks that might be necessary to build the future we want. And if we feel anything even remotely like failure, our instinct may be to run, tail between our legs, back to the security of the life that we had previously decided did not make us happy. There must be a middle ground somewhere between living through failure after failure and never even try-ing. That middle ground is made possible by careful planning, calculated risk-taking, and tenacity. Lots of tenacity.

So, bearing all this in mind, consider it a given that most people will not understand or value your *true* progress toward living out your goals. Save any discussion of this deeply per-sonal truth for your mentor, or for friends/peers with whom you have an understanding or agreement about such things. Or, talk only to yourself about your goals! You can carry on a very interesting dialogue right in your own head! Come on ... we do it all the time. Remember all that negative self-talk? Intentional, positive self-talk is a transformative way to build inner trust and knowingness. If you are shy about talking to yourself, you can write in a journal or diary. No matter how you do it, monitoring and evaluating your progress by periodically checking in with yourself and your feelings is an important aspect of continuing your growth and sense of success.

One thing I learned about while working on this book is the power of containment. In the initial stages of work, I talked to everyone, it seemed, about the book I was going to write. Probably out of my own fear that this was a project I could not or would not actually complete, their validation was something I needed. As the work progressed, I began to realize that every time I discussed it with people, they gave me their feedback (which, of course, I was indirectly asking for), and it became harder for me to simply work toward my goal without being distracted by what everyone else thought about nurses and careers and goals and the price of tea in China.

It took a conscious effort for me to stop this pattern. A *very* conscious effort. And in the process, I came to understand a lifelong pattern I'd had: needing to talk about everything I was thinking and doing. It is not unusual for people to seek this type of validation. What I had never realized is how the very process of seeking validation led to increased pressure and anxiety, because now it had been spoken *out loud*. So now I couldn't change my mind because I might be seen as a "flake" … and the mind raced on, the inner critic and saboteur running rampant. There is a lot to be said for containing this entire process within yourself. Listen to yourself. Support yourself. Allow yourself to make your own journey, follow your intuitions and whims. After all, no one else can tell you how you'll know when you get there … and, the conundrum of it all is that there really is no *"there"* to get, anyway!

Perhaps the best we can hope for is the inner knowing that our actions are in alignment with our values and goals. Maybe *this* is the true meaning of success! I imagine this sense of knowing is different for everyone, but for me there is a very distinct physical sense of alignment, or rightness, when things are true for me. Usually a strong feeling of happiness, joy, or contentment comes over me. Or it may feel like a lifting in my heart; sort of like excitement. There is also a very distinct, unsettled feeling that comes when I'm choosing to do something that I don't want to or that isn't right for me. Sometimes it is a sinking feeling in my stomach or a catch in my heart or throat. Sometimes it just feels *wrong*, and I couldn't possibly tell you how I know this. Pay attention to these physical signs, called everything from "gut feelings" to "belly faith." Once you become familiar with this inner sense of knowing, you will have a valuable tool to help keep you on track.

HOW CAN YOU CONTINUE TO GROW IN SUCCESS?

To continue to grow in success, we need to be willing to live without a Grand Goal, and keep our goals in perspective. It all comes around, full-circle, back to the change process. It has been said that change is the only constant in the universe. If this is true, then we need to have the flexibility of the *tsunami* surfer mentioned in Chapter 2, riding the ever-changing waves in order to move into the future we desire. We must be willing to invest the time and energy needed to become clear about our achievements, values, and goals—and then be willing to toss them out the window when life hands us a different set of circumstances.

Angeles Arrien, anthropologist and Basque folklore specialist, describes what she calls "the four-fold way." In her article, "Four Basic Archetypal Ways Found in Shamanic Traditions," she cites as a pervasive belief in shamanic societies that life can be very simple if we practice these basic principles:

1. *Show up.* To show up is to be visible, to participate in life, and to empower and inspire others through your example and what you model.

2. *Pay attention.* To pay attention is to become aware of all that is going on around you and to notice what has heart or meaning for you. It is a form of courage, which means the ability "to stand by one's core."

3. *Tell the truth.* To tell the truth without blame or judgment is to maintain authenticity. Telling the truth breaks through patterns of denial and allows us to be fully present with ourselves and each other. It allows us to have satisfying and fulfilling human relationships.

4. *Be open to outcome.* Being open to outcome means you must learn to trust and to be comfortable during the times of not knowing. A form of wisdom, this type of trust asks us to step out of our need for control and *allow* the future to emerge as it may, rather than attempt to *make* the future what we think we want.

Now, these may not be the keys to eternal wisdom or the secrets to a successful life, but I was struck by the profound wisdom and practicality of these principles. They speak to living life fully in the moment. We show up each day when we courageously face whatever life puts in front of us. When we pay attention to what is happening around us, we can ride the waves of change and come into sync with the rhythms of life that surround us. When we tell the truth—first and foremost, to ourselves—we pull the process of living close into our hearts and allow it to unfold from the inside out, as a reflection of our true essence. And, when we remain unattached to the outcome, we participate in the miracles of synchronicity, creation, and joy that exist at the core of our nature.

▲ ▲ ▲

These are incredible times. The waves of change that we, as a culture, are currently experiencing seem to issue a challenge for us to be all that we can be. My heartfelt wish is that we will each come to understand the opportunities that exist for us, and then have the courage and confidence to step forward, take action, and live as we dream.

Perhaps, as we learn how to put our fierce courage, vast intelligence, and tender compassion to work for *ourselves* as well as we do for others, we will step into the unknown horizons of the future and discover our great work, our passion in life.

May your life—both professional and personal—be a joyful expression of that passion.

Resource Guide

REFERENCES

Ambrose, Yvonne, RN, CCRN. "Nursing in 2001: Are You Ready?" *Nursing Management*, December 1990: 45-48.

American Nurses Association. *Progress Report on Unlicensed Assistive Personnel.* Report to the House of Delegates, Washington, D.C., 1992.

Ardery, Gail. "Mentors and Protégés: From Ideology to Knowledge," *Current Issues in Nursing*, fourth edition. Iowa City: Mosby, 1994.

Arrien, Angeles. "Four Basic Archetypal Ways Found in Shamanic Traditions," *ReVISION* 13(2), Fall 1990: 59-66.

Aydelotte, Myrtle K. "Entrepreneurs: Issues and Barriers to Independent Practice," *Current Issues in Nursing*, fourth edition. Iowa City: Mosby, 1994.

Bolles, Richard. *The 1996 What Color is Your Parachute? A Practical Manual for Job-Hunters and Career Changers.* Berkeley: Ten Speed Press, 1996.

Bridges, William. *Managing Transitions: Making the Most of Change.* Reading, Massachusetts: Addison-Wesley Publishing Co., 1991.

Buscherhof, Jean R. and Elaine Seymour. "On My Own Terms: The Redefinition of Success in Nursing," *Image: Journal of Nursing Scholarship* 22(2), Spring 1990: 84-88.

Carlson, Kathy, RN, BSN, CPAN. "Change," *Journal of Post-Anesthesia Nursing* 4(2), April 1989:137-138.

Chinn, Peggy L. "Where and When Does Change Begin?" *Nursing Outlook* 40(3), May/June 1992: 102-103.

Curran, Connie R. "An Interview with Karlene M. Kerfoot," *Nursing Economic$*, May-June 1991: 141-147.

Daniels, L. Ann, M.Ed. "Developing Effective Change Agents," *Hospital Topics*, January/February 1986: 32-39.

Davis, Peter S., MA, DEd(Hons), CertEd, SRN, DipN, ONC. "The Meaning of Change to Individuals Within a College of Nurse Education," *Journal of Advanced Nursing*, January 1991: 108-115.

Defeo, Daniel J., RN, MA. "Change: A Central Concern of Nursing," *Nursing Science Quarterly*, Summer 1990: 88-94.

Estela, Linda. *Alternative Careers in Nursing*. Hayward, California: Nurses Research Publications, 1995.

Eubanks, Paula. "Long-Term Career Planning: Flexibility is Key," *Hospitals* 65(21), November 5, 1991:62.

Evans, S. Ann, RN, MS, MBA. "The Noah Principle: Change, Challenge, and Creativity," *Heart and Lung* 19(4), July 1990: 23A-25A.

Goertz Koerner, JoEllen, RN, MS, FAAN and Sandra Schmidt Bunkers, RN, MS. "Transformational Leadership: The Power of Symbol," *Nursing Administration Quarterly*, Fall 1992: 1-9.

Grant, Patricia S., BSN, RN, CIC. "Manage Nurse Stress and Increase Potential at the Bedside," *Nursing Administration Quarterly*, Fall 1993: 16-22.

Hammers, Marilyn. "Rehab in the '90s," *NURSEWEEK* 6(20), July 5, 1993: 6-9.

Heim, Pat with Susan K. Golant. *Hardball for Women: Winning at the Game of Business*. Los Angeles: RGA Publishing Group, 1992.

Joel, Lucille A. "Changes Within the Hospital as a Place of Practice," *Current Issues in Nursing*, fourth edition. Iowa City: Mosby, 1994.

Johnson, Debbie, RN, CPAN. "Change Begins with You," *Journal of Post-Anesthesia Nursing* 4(2), April 1989: 67-68.

Kaplan, Susan Mullen. "The Nurse as Change Agent," *Dermatology Nursing*, December 1991: 419-422.

Kellcher, Patricia. "Home Health Care Takes Center Stage," HealthCareReview@mednexus.com, 1996.

Linney, Barbara. "Values: What's Really Important to You?" *Physician Executive* 20(6), June 1994: 41.

Lundeen, Sally Peck. "Nursing Centers: Models for Autonomous Nursing Practice," *Current Issues in Nursing*, fourth edition. Iowa City: Mosby, 1994.

Manion, Jo, RN, MA, CNAA. "The Nurse Intrapreneur: How to Innovate from Within," *American Journal of Nursing* 94(1), January 1994.

_____. "Nurse Intrapreneurs: The Heroes of Health Care's Future," *Nursing Outlook* 39(1), January/February 1991.

Moses, Evelyn, Chief, Nursing Data and Analysis Staff, U.S. Department of Health and Human Services, Division of Nursing. Information from the 1992 survey of nurses.

Muller-Smith, Patricia, RN, EdD. "Managing from the Neutral Zone," *Journal of Post-Anesthesia Nursing* 8(4), August 1993: 290-292.

New Jersey Department of Health. *A Prospective Reimbursement System Based on Patient Case Mix for New Jersey Hospitals*, 1976-1983. Second annual report, vol. 1. Trenton, New Jersey: State of New Jersey Department of Health, 1978.

Ogilvy, James. *Living Without a Goal: Finding the Freedom to Live a Creative and Innovative Life*. New York: Doubleday, 1995.

Perlman, Dottie and George Takacs. "The 10 Stages of Change," *Nursing Management*, April 1990: 33-38.

Phillips-Jones, Linda. *The New Mentors and Protégés: How to Succeed with the New Mentoring Partnerships*. Grass Valley, California: Coalition of Counseling Centers, 1993.

Rider, Anne C., RGN, RM, MTD. "Being Creative with Change," *Midwives Chronicle & Nursing Notes*, May 1991: 150-151.

RoAne, Susan. *How to Work a Room*. New York: Warner Books, 1988.

Sandroff, Ronni. "The Psychology of Change," *Working Woman*, July 1993: 52-56.

Schorr, Thelma M., RN. "Nurse-Run Managed Care?" *American Journal of Nursing* 90(10), October 1990: 25.

Schweitzer, Jane, RN, MPA. *Tears and Rage: The Nursing Crisis in America*. Fair Oaks, California: Adams-Blake Publishing, 1996.

Scott, Cecelia B. and Linda Moneyham. "Perceptions of Senior Residents about a Community-Based Nursing Center," *IMAGE: Journal of Nursing Scholarship* 27(3), Fall 1995.

Shames, Karilee Halo. *The Nightengale Conspiracy*, revised second edition. Montclair, New Jersey: Enlightenment Press, 1993.

Sheehan, John, Msc, Med, DepFE, RGN, RMN, FRSH. "Investigating Change in a Nursing Context," *Journal of Advanced Nursing*, July 1990: 819-824.

Spina, Vicki. *Getting Hired in the '90s*. Chicago: Dearborn Financial Publishing, 1995.

Styles, Margretta. *On Specialization in Nursing: Toward a New Empowerment.* Washington, D.C.: American Nurses Publishers, 1989.

Swan, John, RMN, RGn and Bob MacVicar, RMN, RGN, BscNurs, MSc. "The Rough Guide to Change," *Nursing Times* 88(13), March 25, 1992: 48-49.

Turner, Susan Odegaard, RN, MBA, MN. "Laid Off? Now What?" *Nursing95,* May 1995: 94-98.

U.S. Bureau of the Census, *Statistical Abstract of the United States:* 1995, 115th edition. Washington, D.C.: U.S. Government Printing Office, 1995.

U.S. Bureau of Labor Statistics, *Occupational Outlook Handbook,* 90-91.Washington, D.C.: U.S. Government Printing Office, 1992.

U.S. Bureau of Labor Statistics, *Occupational Outlook Quarterly* 30(3), Fall 1986.

Vance, C. "Women Leaders: Modern Day Heroines or Societal Deviants?" *Image: Journal of Nursing Scholarship* 11(2), 1979: 37.

Vogel, Gerry and Nancy Doleysh. *Entrepreneuring: A Nurse's Guide to Starting a Business.* New York: National League for Nursing, 1988.

Welton, John M., RN, MSN. "Going Into Business as a Nurse," *American Journal of Nursing,* December 1989.

Winwood, Richard I. *Time Management: An Introduction to the Franklin System.* Salt Lake City, Utah: Franklin International Institute, 1990.

Zimmerman, Polly Gerber. "10 Tips for a Top Interview," *Nursing95,* September 1995: 83-87.

SAMPLE RESUME

MaryAnn Stimpson
1356 First Ave. SW
Tallahassee, FL   55738   883-746-2239

SUMMARY/HIGHLIGHTS

Well-rounded problem-solver with broad base of clinical experience and leadership abilities.
- Delivered expert nursing care to patients in pediatrics setting for over 15 years.
- Developed and implemented preceptor training module for newly graduated nurses.
- Managed all operational aspects of pediatrics unit, including staffing, delegation of duties, direct supervision, team-building, and quality control.
- Developed and taught continuing education programs on leadership, change, and stress.

PROFESSIONAL HISTORY

University Medical Center, Miami, FL   4/92 to present
Staff Nurse IV, Pediatrics, PICU

Perform duties as charge nurse, clinical team member, and act as professional resource for staff.
- Developed and implemented new emergency policies and procedures for pediatric patients.
- Streamlined charting guidelines, resulting in a 60% reduction in staff overtime.
- Performed annual educational needs analyses and planned 1994-1996 educational agenda.
- Organized and facilitated classes for staff on a variety of topics, including respiratory care, central lines and monitoring, emergency review, blood gas analysis, and electrolytes.

Develop and teach continuing education courses on stress, burnout, change management, and leadership.
- Courses offered hospital-wide, twice a year, through the education department.
- Taught most highly attended class (Leadership for Nurses) three years in a row.

St. John's Medical Center, Austin, TX   8/83 to 4/88
Staff Nurse III, Pediatric Oncology

Provided team-based patient care to patients on a busy pediatric oncology unit.

EDUCATION

Baccalaureate of Science in Nursing, Texas University, Austin, TX.   6/83
- Graduated with academic honors.
- Served on curriculum committee for two years.

REFERENCES

Available upon request

SAMPLE RESUME

Jane R. Smith
1818 Woodford Place
Smithson, NC 44980
Home phone: 770-555-3242

OBJECTIVE
To work in education, training, and/or product demonstration.

QUALIFICATIONS
Have worked as an RN for 18 years in critical care. Significant experience in teaching and training, and a long-standing interest in medical equipment and supplies.

WORK HISTORY

RN, St. Agnes Medical Center, Jonesville, NC   12/79 to present
CCRN, ICU & Cardiopulmonary Unit, Clinical Staff Nurse III and IV for 7 years.
Committees:
- Product Evaluation (10 years). Selected, evaluated, and provided in-service training for new products to staff throughout the hospital.
- Professional Nursing Board of Review.
- PPC (Professional Performance Committee).
Teaching:
- Precepted many students and new staff for more than 16 years.
- Developed classes for staff RNs on how to be preceptors.
- Taught classes on cardiac surgery, hemodynamic monitoring, and bedside patient monitoring for students and new staff
Projects:
- Radiation Oncology Resource Book. Collected and edited resources.
- ICU/CPU Reference Book. Helped codify hospital standards, collected and edited resources.
- Published a hospital-wide nursing newsletter during a hospital merger.

RN, Doctors Hospital, Asheville, NC   6/78 to 12/79
- Worked in medical, surgical, and intensive care units.

EDUCATION

St. Jude's Hospital School of Nursing, Charlottesville, NC   4/75 to 6/78
Nursing diploma. Eleanor Higby Memorial Award for most outstanding all-around student in clinical nursing and theory.

North Carolina University, Asheville, NC   8/67 to 6/69
Liberal Arts

VOLUNTEER ACTIVITY

Heart-to-Heart International Children's Medical Alliance   10/91 to 11/95
Helped establish an adult open-heart surgery program at a hospital in St. Petersburg, Russia. Over a five-year period, helped solicit and collect several million dollars worth of equipment and supplies donated by American companies. Was a key participant in a medical training team that made three trips to Russia to train nurses and doctors.

REFERENCES
Available upon request

SAMPLE RESUME – NEW GRADUATE

JANET MARIE JONES
1515 Hayes Street ✧ Toledo ✧ Ohio ✧ 90909 ✧ 490-555-8834

HIGHLIGHTS / SUMMARY: Recent graduate of University of Cleveland School of Nursing with four years of experience as a nursing assistant, excellent clinical skills developed during clinical rotations, and a highly enthusiastic, positive attitude.

EDUCATION:
University of Cleveland School of Nursing, **Cleveland, Ohio**
Bachelor of Science in Nursing, June 1996
Licensed Registered Nurse: Ohio

Course work included public health policy; independent study project in the Sexual Assault Resource Center, Cleveland County Hospital; research paper on clinical complications of hysterectomies.

Significant clinical rotations:
St. Agnes's Middle School Girls' Health Clinic: Senior Leadership Clinical
VA Medical Center, Cleveland: Medical/surgical; special focus on respiratory illnesses
Children's Hospital of Cleveland: Medical/surgical pediatrics
University Hospital of Cleveland: Cardiac intensive care and step-down
VA Medical Center: Psychiatric/mental health
VNA of Cleveland: Community health
St. Mary's Hospital, Cleveland: Maternal/child health

WORK EXPERIENCE:
University Hospital of Cleveland, **Cleveland, Ohio**   **Nursing Assistant. 10/92 - 7/96**
Responsible for providing patient care to medical/surgical patients as directed by staff nurse. Served on new-hire training committee and participated in the development of preceptor training program for med/surg department.

Southside YMCA, **Cleveland, Ohio**   **Senior Lifeguard. 4/83 - 10/92**
Taught swimming lessons to children, ages 6 months to 12 years. Coached city swim team. Provided private swimming lessons. Served as lifeguard during summer months.

Girl Scouts of America, **Cleveland, Ohio**   **Summer Camp Counselor. 6/82 - 9/82**
Coordinated activities, taught first-aid courses, and promoted self-confidence and self-awareness. Conducted discussion groups with young girls, ages 8 to 12.

ADDITIONAL INFORMATION:
Was voted "Best Clinical Resource" by graduating nursing class, June 1996.
Interested in pursuing career in women's health arena.

REFERENCES:
Available on request

LETTER OF INTRODUCTION
INFORMATIONAL INTERVIEW

MaryAnn Stimpson
1356 First Ave. SW
Tallahassee, FL 55738
883-746-2239

February 28, 1997

Ms. Jane Doe
Director
Quality Review, Inc.
Sun City, CA 95554

Dear Ms. Doe:

I recently read a book on career development for nurses, and found myself very interested in making a career change into Utilization Review and/or Quality Assurance. It was suggested that talking with someone in the field of UR/QA could be an excellent way for me to gather information to assist me in my decision-making process.

Your position as director of Quality Review Incorporated clearly indicates your success in this industry. Meeting with you to obtain your insights and opinions on QA/UR would be a tremendous help to me in planning this transition.

Please understand that I do not expect you to know of any permanent or temporary opportunities at this time. Rather, our meeting would provide me a better understanding of what is happening in your industry.

Enclosed is a summary of my background outlining my strengths and accomplishments, which will give you an idea of my work experience. I will call you early next week to ask if it would be convenient for us to meet, and, if so, to arrange a short appointment (15 to 20 minutes) at a mutually convenient time.

I look forward to talking with you!

Sincerely,

MaryAnn Stimpson

LETTER OF INTRODUCTION
INFORMATIONAL INTERVIEW – NEW GRADUATE

JANET MARIE JONES
1515 Hayes Street ◇ Toledo ◇ Ohio ◇ 90909 ◇ 490-555-8834

March 12, 1997

Ms. Nancy Nurse
Nurse Recruiter
ABC Medical Center
Augusta, GA 49496

Dear Ms. Nurse:

As a recent graduate from the University of Cleveland School of Nursing, I have a great interest in current hiring trends for the nursing profession. Helen Huber at the School of Nursing suggested that I contact you as a source of information about this rapidly changing field. Meeting with you to discuss the future of nursing as it relates to *my* future as a nurse would be extremely helpful to me as I plan my career.

Please understand that I do not expect you to either have a position or know of any positions for me. Rather, our discussion would provide me with information and advice on how to develop my career in nursing.

Enclosed, please find my résumé. This outlines my background and experience, and will give you some idea of my strengths and accomplishments. I will call you early next week to see if it is convenient for you to meet with me. If so, we could arrange a short, 15- to 20-minute meeting at a mutually convenient time.

I look forward to talking with you next week!

Sincerely,

Janet Jones

THANK-YOU LETTER
INFORMATIONAL INTERVIEW

MaryAnn Stimpson
1356 First Ave. SW
Tallahassee, FL 55738
883-746-2239

January 14, 1997

Ms. Jane Doe
Director
Quality Review Inc.
Sun City, CA 95554

Dear Jane:

Thank you for taking time out of your busy schedule to talk with me this morning about the Quality Assurance and Utilization Review industry. The information you provided is invaluable, and your suggestions are very helpful in my efforts to redirect my career. I especially value the insight you provided into the preparatory courses available that can facilitate my entry into this field.

As you suggested, I will contact your associate, Jane Brown, for additional information on how a nurse with critical care experience can best make this transition. And, using the catalog you gave me, I will begin selecting classes today!

It was a pleasure to meet you. As we discussed, I will keep you apprised of my progress in this endeavor.

Sincerely,

MaryAnn Stimpson

THANK-YOU LETTER
INFORMATIONAL INTERVIEW – NEW GRADUATE

JANET MARIE JONES
1515 Hayes Street ◇ Toledo ◇ Ohio ◇ 90909 ◇ 490-555-8834

March 19, 1997

Ms. Nancy Nurse
Nurse Recruiter
ABC Medical Center
Augusta, GA 49496

Dear Nancy:

Thank you so much for taking the time to talk with me this morning about the future hiring trends of the nursing profession. The time we spent together was invaluable, and the very practical information you shared with me about the typical hiring process will be a great help as I pursue a job in nursing.

I especially appreciate your feedback and insight into the areas of nursing that would best match the characteristics of my personality and background. Finding the "right" job is a priority to me, and your perspective in this arena was both thought-provoking and motivating.

As you suggested, I will contact Mary Johnson at XYZ Medical Center about the new Women's Health Center she is opening this fall. I look forward to meeting with her!

Thank you again. I will, as we discussed, let you know how things go with Ms. Johnson.

Sincerely,

Janet Jones

COVER LETTER

MaryAnn Stimpson
1356 First Ave. SW
Tallahassee, FL 55738
883-746-2239

February 19, 1997

Ms. Belinda Doyle
Senior Clinical Specialist
Healthtronic, Inc.
1280 West 8th Street, #B9-512
Newport News, VA 66560

Dear Ms. Doyle:

It was with great interest and excitement that I read your advertisement for a clinical in-service coordinator in *NURSEWEEK* magazine (March 4th edition). In the seven years that I have worked in critical care nursing, Healthtronic has *always* been recognized as the leading manufacturer of cardiac pacemakers and defibrillator devices, well respected by the doctors and nurses with whom I work.

Functioning in the critical care setting and using your equipment on a daily basis has given me a broad understanding of how your products work. This knowledge, combined with my background as unit preceptor and trainer, allows me to offer a unique service to your corporation. Solid clinical skills, along with a passion for teaching and an independent, entrepreneurial approach to nursing are all qualities that I bring to my work.

Please find enclosed my résumé for your consideration. I look forward to talking with you and gathering more information on Healthtronic's clinical programs. I will call you next week to set up an appointment at a mutually convenient time.

Sincerely,

MaryAnn Stimpson

COVER LETTER

Anna Devenchenzie
1414 Forest View Lane
Ione, FL 49584
748-294-8892

October 3, 1997

Ms. Mae Salter
Home Hospice Nurses of America
4567 5th St.
Ione, FL 49584

Dear Ms. Salter:

As an experienced oncology nurse, I have worked with many patients and families as they move through the death-and-dying process. It was in that setting that I first encountered the hospice movement and developed an interest in working as a home hospice nurse. Home Hospice Nurses of America has a reputation for providing impeccable care to both its clients *and* staff, a fact I have seen demonstrated again and again as my path crosses the paths of the people your work has touched.

In my ten years in oncology, I have developed the clinical and emotional skills required to work in what can be a very demanding setting — and have flourished, thoroughly enjoying the challenge and the rewards. As the next step in my career, I would like to put my considerable knowledge and skills to use in a less intervention-based setting that would allow me to participate actively in death as one of life's great transitions.

My résumé is enclosed for your consideration. I would welcome the opportunity to meet with you to discuss possible job openings at Home Hospice Nurses of America. I am available for an interview at your convenience, and will call your office next week to see if we can arrange a time to meet.

I look forward to speaking with you!

Sincerely,

Anna Devenchenzie

COVER LETTER – NEW GRADUATE

JANET MARIE JONES
1515 Hayes Street ◇ **Toledo** ◇ **Ohio** ◇ **90909** ◇ **490-555-8834**

January 30, 1997

Ms. Mary Martin
Clinical Coordinator
Women's Healthcare Clinic
3456 Maiden Lane
Cleveland, OH 84856

Dear Ms. Martin:

I am writing to introduce myself to you as a recent graduate of the University of Cleveland School of Nursing. I am extremely interested in exploring employment opportunities with the Women's Healthcare Clinic. My interest in women's health has spanned many years, and many of my life experiences and educational pursuits are related to these issues.

As indicated on my enclosed résumé, I have worked with girls/women in arenas ranging from the Girl Scouts to teen health clinics to adult hysterectomy patients. These experiences, along with an excellent maternal/child health clinical rotation at St. Mary's Hospital, have provided me with a broad base of understanding on issues of women's health. This understanding, combined with the clinical experience gained in four years as a nurses' aide, has prepared me to become a highly functional team member, able to contribute to the care of your patients in the manner you so clearly require of your staff.

I would be delighted to begin my career as a registered nurse at Women's Healthcare Clinic. Please give my résumé careful consideration. I will contact you early next week to see if we can arrange a mutually convenient time to discuss employment possibilities at your clinic. If you prefer, you may contact me at 455-766-9345.

I look forward to speaking with you!

Sincerely,

Janet Jones

THANK-YOU LETTER – JOB INTERVIEW

JANE R. ADAMS

5656 Mayfield Lane, Tooley Valley, MD 77456
455-732-8889

September 6, 1997

Ms. Janet Delgado
Manager, IV Therapy Division
Home Health Care of America
14 SW First St.
Dalton, IA 73022

Dear Janet:

Thank you so much for taking the time to meet with me today and discuss the Clinical IV Specialist position at Home Health Care of America. I found our conversation to be very interesting, and am intrigued by some of the new programs you will be implementing this fall—especially the program for pediatric oncology patients.

It is exciting for me to realize that there are companies, such as Home Health Care of America, that are designing programs for home-based oncology care of children which meet or even exceed the standards of care delivered in the hospital setting. Putting over seven years of pediatric oncology experience to work in the home setting will allow me to combine excellent clinical skills with one of my highest priorities: fostering individual growth and independence for the child with cancer. Years of patient and family teaching, care planning and support, along with a compassionate understanding of the ordeal of cancer, provide me with a strong foundation to make an important contribution to your company.

It was a pleasure meeting with you today, and I look forward to hearing from you early next week to further discuss the Clinical IV Specialist position.

Sincerely,

Jane Adams

ACCEPTANCE LETTER

Anna Devenchenzie
1414 Forest View Lane
Ione, FL 49584
748-294-8892

November 14, 1997

Ms. Mae Salter
Home Hospice Nurses of America
4567 5th St.
Ione, FL 49584

Dear Mae:

I am extremely excited to be joining Home Hospice Nurses of America as a staff nurse. Based on our conversation at the interview I feel confident that this will be a challenging and stimulating environment in which to continue my career.

As per our discussion, I understand the salary for this position is $38,000. I will begin work on December 1, 1997, and appreciate your understanding my need to keep the commitments I have made for the week of December 19 through 26.

I look forward to seeing you on December 1!

Sincerely,

Anna Devenchenzie

GENERAL RESOURCES

▲ *Calenders/planners*

Franklin Quest Co. — This is a comprehensive, easy-to-use planning system. It is available by calling the company in Salt Lake City, Utah (800-654-1776), and in retail centers located in some of the larger malls. Franklin markets a full array of products (including books, audio/videotapes, seminars, etc.) to assist you in setting up and fully utilizing the system.

The Seven Habits Executive/Pocket Organizer — This system was designed by Steven Covey, author of the bestseller *The Seven Habits of Highly Effective People.* It is complemented by an array of optional audio/video and written material to get you on your way. You can order the Executive/pocket organizer from the Covey Leadership Center in Provo, Utah (800-553-8889).

Day Timer — Another comprehensive system which allows you to add the sections, such as goal planning, that you want to use. It is available in some office supply stores, or by calling 800-225-5005.

Day Runner — This planning system has been around a long time, and is available in many department and stationery stores. You can call for a catalog, if you prefer (800-635-5544).

▲ *Magazines*

There are numerous magazines and journals available for nurses. Check your local or hospital library for a complete listing. Also, refer to the nursing organizations listed at the end of this section for additional specialty-specific publications. Here are some popular nursing magazines and contact information for ordering them.

Heart & Lung: The Journal of Critical Care. $36/year.
Journal Subscription Services
Mosby—Year Book, Inc.
11830 Westline Industrial Dr.
St. Louis, MO 63146-3318
800-453-4351
314-872-8370

IMAGE: The Journal of Nursing Scholarship. $16/year.
IMAGE Publication Office
Sigma Theta Tau International
   Society for Nursing
550 W. North St.
Indianapolis, IN 46202
888-634-7575
317-634-8171

RN. $35/year.
Circulation Department
P.O. Box 57140
Boulder, CO 80322-7140
800-284-8945

Revolution: The Journal of Nurse Empowerment. $24.95/year.
A.D. Von Publishers, Inc.
56 McArthur Ave.
Staten Island, NY 10312
800-967-2961
718-948-4938

NURSEWEEK
Circulation Department
1156-C Aster Ave.
Sunnyvale, CA 94086-6801
800-221-5946
408-249-5877

Nursing. $42/year.
Nursing
1111 Bethlehem Pike
P.O. Box 908
Springhouse, PA 19477
215-646-8700

Moving Network - Call 800-777-0919 for information on:

California—*NURSEWEEK*

Delaware—*The Nursing Spectrum*

District of Columbia—*The Nursing Spectrum*

Florida—*The Nursing Spectrum*

Illinois—*The Nursing Spectrum*

Kansas—*Kansas City Nursing News*

Maryland—*The Nursing Spectrum*

Massachusetts—*Boston Nurse News*

Michigan—*RN Excellence*

Missouri—*Kansas City Nursing News*

New Jersey—*The Nursing Spectrum*

New York—*The Nursing Spectrum*

North Carolina—*Nursing Matters*

Ohio—*Nursing News* (Cleveland)

Pennsylvania—*The Nursing Spectrum* (Philadelphia)
Nursing News (Pittsburgh)

Texas—*NURSEWEEK*

Virginia—*The Nursing Spectrum* (D.C. Metro)
Nursing Matters (Southern Virginia)

Wisconsin—*Nursing Matters*

NURSING ORGANIZATIONS

▲ *Alternative/spiritual organizations*

American Holistic Nurses Association (AHNA)
  4101 Lake Boone Trail, Suite 201
  Raleigh, NC 27607
  919-787-5181, fax: 919-787-4916
Objectives are to: promote education for nurses and the public on the concept of holistic health care; examine new directions of health care delivery, especially within nursing; serve as a network for persons interested in holistic nursing. Offers an annual conference. Publications: *Beginnings*, monthly newsletter, included in membership dues, $16/year for non-members; *Journal of Holistic Nursing*, quarterly, included in membership dues, $28.80/year for non-members.

Anthroposophical Nurses Association of America (ANAA)
  103 Hermitage Dr.
  Elkton, MD 21921
  410-392-3942, fax: 410-392-0862
  Dues: $50/year
Seeks to further the practice of anthroposophical nursing in the United States. Anthroposophy is a 20th-century religious system centering on human development. Encourages nurses to apply their knowledge of humankind to nursing practices. Promotes members' continued education. Holds an annual conference. Publications: Annual newsletter.

National Association of Nurse Massage Therapists (NANMT)
  P.O. Box 1150
  Abita Springs, LA 70420
  888-462-6686, 504-892-6990, fax: 504-892-7540
  Dues: $75/year, $35/year for students
Promotes the integration of massage and other therapeutic forms of bodywork into existing health care practice. Promotes

nurse massage therapists as specialists within the nursing profession. Sponsors periodic Celebrate! The Magic of Touch conferences. Publications: *Nurse's Touch*, quarterly magazine, included in membership dues.

▲ *Business/leadership organizations*

American Association of Legal Nurse Consultants (AALNC)
  4700 W. Lake Ave.
  Glenview, IL 60025-1485
  847-375-4713, fax: 847-375-4777
  Dues: $85/year
Promotes professional advancement of registered nurses consulting within the legal arena by providing a forum for education and exchange of information. Conducts annual educational program. Holds an annual conference and seminar. Publications: *The Journal of Legal Nurse Consulting*, quarterly, included in membership dues.

American Medical Writers Association (AMWA)
  9650 Rockville Pike
  Bethesda, MD 20814
  301-493-0003, fax: 301-493-6384
  Dues: $75
Objectives are to: bring together into one association individuals who are interested in any aspect of communication in the medical and allied scientific professions; promote standards of excellence in biomedical communications, and inform and encourage all those interested in improving the quality and effectiveness of biomedical communications; provide educational opportunities that lead to, support, and enhance excellence in medical communication. Holds an annual conference and regional workshops.

American Organization of Nurse Executives (AONE)
  One N. Franklin, 34th Floor
  Chicago, IL 60606
  312-422-2800, fax: 312-422-4503
  Dues: $200/year
Provides leadership, professional development, advocacy, and
research to advance nursing practice and patient care, promote
nursing leadership and excellence, and shape health care public
policy. Offers placement service though career development and
referral center. Holds annual conference. Publications: *AONE
News,* quarterly newsletter, included in membership dues;
AONE Updates, newsletter, included in membership dues.

American Business Women's Association (ABWA)
  9100 Ward Pkwy.
  P.O. Box 8728
  Kansas City, MO 64114-0728
  816-361-6621, fax: 816-361-4991
Provides opportunities for businesswomen to help themselves
and others grow personally and professionally through leadership, education, networking support, and national recognition.
Offers leadership training and discounted CareerTrack programs, a résumé service, credit card and member loan programs,
and travel and insurance benefits. Sponsors American Business
Women's Day and American Business Women's Strut annually
on September 22. Publications: *CONNECT,* monthly newsletter, free to chapter officers, or $7/year; *The Leadership Edge,*
bimonthly newsletter, free to chapter officers, or $10/year.

Carondelet Management Institute
  2090 N. Kolb Rd.
  Tucson, AZ 85715
  800-726-3888, fax: 520-721-3985
Offers CEU classes on medical-legal nursing.

Medical-Legal Consulting Institute, Inc.
  2476 Bolsover, Suite 632
  Houston, TX 77005
  713-961-3078, fax: 713-840-7150
Call or write for free information on courses and products.

National Association of Traveling Nurses (NATN)
  P.O. Box 417-120
  Chicago, IL 60641-7120
  708-453-0080, fax: 708-453-0083
  Dues: $25/year
Provides travel information; offers substantial discounts for members at major hotels, resorts, and car rental agencies. Provides members with complete list of approved travel industry suppliers, including travel agents, vendors, airlines, cruise ship companies, and hotels. Holds annual conference and convention. Publications: *Journal of Traveling Nurses,* quarterly, $2.95/issue.

National Nurses in Business Association (NNBA)
  56 McArthur Ave.
  Staten Island, NY 10312
  800-331-6534, fax: 718-317-0858
Serves as support group for nurses interested in seeking business opportunities. Provides business-related information, sponsors speakers' bureau, offers placement service. Offers access to a 1-800-HELPLINE and 1-800-RESOURCE HOTLINE for member consultation, counsel, and referral services. Runs annual conference. Publications: *Revolution — The Journal of Nurse Empowerment,* quarterly journal, included in membership dues.

Small Business Association
  P.O. Box 1000
  Fort Worth, TX 76119
  800-827-5722

The SBA has offices throughout the country. Consult the U.S. government section in your telephone directory for the office nearest you. SBA offers a number of programs and services, including training and educational programs, counseling services, financial programs, and contract assistance. Ask about the Service Corps of Retired Executives (SCORE), a national organization of volunteers who provide free counseling, workshops, and seminars to prospective and existing small business owners. Small Business Development Centers (SBDCs) are sponsored by the SBA in partnership with state and local governments, the educational community, and the private sector. They provide assistance, counseling and training to prospective and existing small business people. Small Business Institutes (SBIs) are organized through the SBA on more than 500 college campuses nationwide. The institutes provide counseling by students and faculty to small business owners. Publications: The SBA offers numerous books, pamphlets, and brochures for a nominal fee.

▲ *Community/public health organizations*

American Public Health Association (APHA)
    1015 15th St. NW, Suite 300
    Washington, D.C. 20005
    202-789-5600, fax: 202-789-5661
Seeks to protect and promote personal, mental, and environmental health. Services include promulgation of standards, establishment of uniform practices and procedures, research on the etiology of communicable diseases, research in public health, and exploration of medical care programs and their relationship to public health. Holds annual American Public Health Association Meeting. Publications: *American Journal of Public Health,* monthly, included in membership dues, $80/year for non-members; *The Nation's Health,* 10 issues/year, included in membership dues, $8/year for non-members.

International Conference on Community Health Centers
  1801 Meison Neuve W., Room 600
  H3H1J9 Montreal, Canada
  514-842-9500
Over 15 health care providers from 35 countries. Conducts workshops, oral presentations. Promotes the role of member organizations, assists in the development of new centers, while respecting each center's unique personality.

▲ *Educational organizations*

American Association for Cancer Education (AACE)
  c/o Robert M. Chamberlain
  M. D. Anderson Cancer Center
  Dept. of Epidemiology, Box 189
  1515 Holcombe Blvd.
  Houston, TX 77030
  713-792-3020, fax: 713-792-0807
Provides a forum for physicians, dentists, nurses, health educators, social workers, and occupational therapists concerned with the study and improvement of cancer education focusing on prevention, early detection, treatment, and rehabilitation.

American Association of Diabetes Educators (AADE)
  444 N. Michigan Ave., Suite 1240
  Chicago, IL 60611-3901
  800-338-DMED, 312-644-2233, fax: 312-644-4411
  Dues: $75/year
Purposes are to provide educational opportunities for the professional growth and development of members, promote the development of quality diabetes education for the diabetic consumer, foster communication and cooperation among individuals and organizations involved in diabetes patient education, and offer continuing education programs for diabetes educators.

Holds AADE Annual Meeting and Educational Program every August. Publications: *AADE News,* 9 issues/year, newsletter, included in membership dues; *The Diabetes Educator,* bimonthly journal, included in membership dues, $45 for non-members.

American Association for Health Education (AAHE)
    1900 Association Dr.
    Reston, VA 20191-1599
    703-476-3437, fax: 703-476-6638
    Dues: $100
For professionals responsible for health education in schools, colleges, communities, hospitals, clinics, and industries. Holds an annual meeting. Publications: *HE-Extra,* 6 issues/year, included in membership dues; *Journal of Health Education,* bimonthly.

American Cancer Society (ACS)
    1599 Clifton Rd. NE
    Atlanta, GA 30329
    800-ACS-2345, 404-320-3333, fax: 404-325-0230
Supports education and research in cancer prevention, diagnosis, detection, and treatment. Provides special services to cancer patients. Sponsors Reach to Recovery, CanSurmount, and I Can Cope. Conducts medical and educational programs.

American Heart Association (AHA)
    7272 Greenville Ave.
    Dallas, TX 75231-4596
    800-242-1793, 214-373-6300
Supports research, education, and community service programs with the objective of reducing premature death and disability from cardiovascular diseases and stroke; coordinates the efforts of physicians, nurses, health professionals, and others engaged in the fight against heart and circulatory disease.

American Society for Training and Development (ASTD)
    1640 King St., Box 1443
    Alexandria, VA   22313-2043
    703-683-8100
Provides leadership to individuals interested in training and communication. Publications: *Training and Development Magazine,* monthly, $85/year; *Technical and Skills Training,* 8 issues/year, $59/year; *Human Resource Development Quarterly,* quarterly journal, $79/year; numerous other publications available to members.

Mended Hearts (MH)
    7272 Greenville Ave.
    Dallas, TX   75231-4596
    214-706-1442, fax: 214-987-4334
Works to provide advice, encouragement, and services to heart disease patients and their families. Holds an annual conference. Publications: *Heartbeat,* quarterly.

National Center for Health Education (NCHE)
    72 Spring St., Suite 208
    New York, NY   10012-4019
    212-334-9470, fax: 212-334-9845
For professionals promoting health education in schools, communities, and family settings. Aims to "extend the reach and power of education for health." Advocates health education and health promotion; builds coalitions of private and public sector groups; documents, develops, and disseminates model programs. Manages Growing Healthy, a comprehensive school health education curriculum. Holds periodic conferences and seminars.

Society for Public Health Education (SOPHE)
    1015 15th St. NW, Suite 410
    Washington, D.C.   20005
    202-408-9804, fax: 202-408-9815

Seeks to promote, encourage, and contribute to the advancement of health for all people by encouraging study, improving health practices, and elevating standards of achievement in public health education. Holds annual meeting, in conjunction with the American Public Health Association. Publications: *Health Education Quarterly*, quarterly newsletter.

▲ Home care/hospice organizations

Hospice Nurses Association (HNA)
    Medical Center East
    211 N. Whitfield St., Suite 375
    Pittsburgh, PA 15206
    412-361-2470, fax: 412-361-2425
    Dues: $45/year, $25/year for students

Promotes high professional standards in hospice nursing. Conducts education and research programs. Has a certification process. Holds periodic meetings. Publications: *Fanfare*, quarterly newsletter.

National Association for Home Care (NAHC)
    228 7th St. SE
    Washington, D.C. 20003
    202-547-7425, fax: 202-547-3540

Develops and promotes high standards of patient care in home care services. Sponsors educational programs for organizations and individuals. Seeks to affect legislative and regulatory processes concerning home care services, gathers and disseminates home care industry data, develops public relations strategies, and works to increase political visibility of home care services. Holds annual meeting and Homecare Expo each fall. Publications: *Homecare News*, monthly tabloid, included in membership dues, $18/year for non-members; *Hospice Forum*, biweekly newsletter, included in membership dues, $105/year for non-members; *NAHC Report*, weekly newsletter, included in membership dues, $325/year for non-members.

Visiting Nurse Associations of America (VNAA)
c/o Pam Hamilton
3801 E. Florida Ave., Suite 900
Denver, CO 80210
888-866-8773, 303-753-0218, fax: 303-753-0258

Develops competitive strength among community-based non-profit visiting nurse organizations, works to strengthen business resources and economic programs through contracting, marketing, governmental affairs, and publications. Sponsors the VNA Annual Meeting.

▲ *Inpatient care/clinical practice organizations*

American Association of Critical-Care Nurses (AACN)
101 Columbia
Aliso Viejo, CA 92656
714-362-2000, fax: 714-362-2020
e-mail: aacninfo@iqnow.org

Serves nurses practicing in the critical care setting. Offers educational workshops and a certification program for critical care nurses. Sponsors the annual National Teaching Institute and Critical Care Expo. Publications: *American Journal of Critical Care*; *Critical Care Nurse*.

American Association of Neuroscience Nurses (AANN)
224 N. Des Plaines, #601
Chicago, IL 60661
800-477-2266, 312-993-0043, fax: 312-993-0362
Dues: $68/year ($34/year for students)

Fosters interest, education, and high standards of practice in the field of neuroscience nursing. Encourages continuing growth in the field, and provides a medium for communication among neuroscience nurses in the U.S. and Canada. Holds an annual conference. Publications: *American Association of Neuro-*

science Nurses Synapse, bimonthly newsletter, included in membership dues; *Journal of Neuroscience Nursing,* bimonthly, included in membership dues, $45/year for non-members.

American Association of Spinal Cord Injury Nurses (AASCIN)
    75-20 Astoria Blvd.
    Jackson Heights, NY 11370-1177
    718-803-3782, ext. 258, fax: 718-803-0414
    Dues: $75/year
Works to promote and improve nursing care of spinal cord injury patients, develop and advance related education and research, and recognize nurses whose careers are devoted to the problems of spinal cord injury patients. Conducts research and educational programs. Holds an annual conference and workshop. Publications: *Education Guide for Spinal Cord Injury Nurses: A Manual for Teaching Patients, Families and Caregivers,* $20; *Spinal Cord Injury: Educational Content for Professional Nursing Practice,* $20; *SCI Nursing,* quarterly journal.

American Board of Post-Anesthesia Nursing Certification (ABPANC)
    475 Riverside Dr., 7th Floor
    New York, NY 10115
    800-622-7262, 212-870-3495, fax: 212-870-3588
Administers examination to individuals wishing to attain post-anesthesia nursing certification. Publications: *CPAN Newsletter,* quarterly, included in membership dues.

American Radiological Nurses Association (ARNA)
    2021 Spring Rd., Suite 600
    Oak Brook, IL 60521
    630-571-9072, fax: 630-571-7837
    Dues: $75/year

Seeks to provide, promote, and maintain quality patient care through education, standards of care, professional growth, and collaboration with other health care providers. Sponsors a semiannual conference. Publications: *Images,* quarterly journal, included in membership dues, $50/year for non-members.

American Society of Post-Anesthesia Nurses (ASPAN)
  9397 Midnight Pass Rd.
  Sarasota, FL 34242-2956
  Fax: 609-848-1881
Promotes upgrading of standards of post-anesthesia patient care and the professional growth of licensed nurses involved in the care of patients in the immediate post-anesthesia period. Conducts courses. Holds an annual meeting/symposium. Publications: *Breathline,* bimonthly newsletter, included in membership dues; *Journal of Postanesthesia Nursing,* bimonthly, included in membership dues, $48/year for non-members.

Association of Operating Room Nurses (AORN)
  2170 S. Parker Rd., Suite 300
  Denver, CO 80231
  800-755-2676, 303-755-6300, fax: 303-750-3212
  Dues: $45/year
Provides education, representation, and standards for quality patient care. Holds annual conference and convention. Publications: *AORN Journal,* monthly, included in membership dues, $50/year for non-members.

Association of Pediatric Oncology Nurses (APON)
  4700 W. Lake Ave.
  Glenview, IL 60025-1485
  847-375-4724, fax: 847-375-4777
  Dues: $65/year, $45/year for students
Scientific and educational association seeking to establish lines of communication among nurses caring for children with

cancer. Encourages updating of literature and development of standards of care. Plans regional workshops. Holds an annual conference. Publications: *APON Newsletter,* quarterly; *Journal of Pediatric Oncology Nursing,* quarterly; *Nursing Care of the Child With Cancer.*

Association of Women's Health, Obstetric, and Neonatal Nurses (AWHONN)
    c/o Communications Department
    700 14th. St. NW, Suite 600
    Washington, D.C. 20005
    202-662-1600, fax: 202-737-0575
Promotes and establishes the highest standards of ob-gyn nursing practice, education, and research; sponsors educational meetings, audiovisual programs, and continuing education courses. Holds regional meetings and an annual research conference. Publications: *Journal of Obstetric, Gynecologic, and Neonatal Nursing,* bimonthly, $26/year, $18/year for students; *NAACOG Newsletter,* monthly, included in membership dues, $5/copy for non-members.

Emergency Nurses Association (ENA)
    216 Higgins Rd.
    Park Ridge, IL 60068
    800-243-8362, 847-698-9400, fax: 847-698-9406
    Dues: $80/year
Objectives are to promote emergency nursing as a profession and establish standards of care in the field, work with other heath-related organizations toward the improvement of emergency care, and serve as a resource for emergency nursing education and research. Holds annual business meeting and annual scientific assembly (with courses and information sessions). Publications: *Etcetera,* newsletter, 9 issues/year; *International Journal of Trauma Nursing,* quarterly; *Journal of Emergency Nursing,* bimonthly.

International Association of Forensic Nurses (IAFN)
    6900 Grove Rd.
    Thorofare, NJ 08086
    609-848-8356, fax: 609-848-5274
    Dues: $75
"Leadership in health care's response to violence." This is the only international professional organization of registered nurses formed exclusively to develop, promote, and disseminate information about the science of forensic nursing. Publications: *On The Edge,* periodic newsletter; *Journal of Forensic Nursing,* to begin publication in 1997.

International Transplant Nurses Society (ITNS)
    Foster Plaza, Bldg. 5
    651 Holiday Dr., Suite 300
    Pittsburgh, PA 15220-2740
    412-928-3667, fax: 412-928-4951
Works to encourage cooperation among all medical disciplines involved in transplantation; disseminate information; and establish certification for this nursing specialty. Holds an annual symposium. Publications: Quarterly newsletter, included in membership dues.

Intravenous Nurses Society (INS)
    Fresh Pond Square
    10 Fawcett St.
    Cambridge, MA 02138
    617-441-3008, fax: 617-441-3009
    Dues: $90
Publications: *Newsline,* bimonthly, included in membership dues; *Journal of Intravenous Nurses,* bimonthly journal.

National Alliance for Infusion Therapy (NAIT)
  1001 Pennsylvania Ave. NW, Suite 600
  Washington, D.C. 20004-2582
  202-347-0066, fax: 202-624-7222
Promotes the appropriate use of infusion therapies (parenteral or enteral administration of drugs or nutrients) at home and in other alternate settings. Seeks to raise awareness of infusion therapies through private payer advocacy of infusion therapy. Establishes and disseminates guidelines for quality patient care. Publications: *Infusion News*, bimonthly newsletter, included in membership dues.

National Association of Neonatal Nurses (NANN)
  1304 Southpoint Blvd., Suite 280
  Petaluma, CA 94954
  707-762-5588, fax: 707-762-0401
  Dues: $50/year
Promotes professional development of members, provides educational and networking opportunities, and disseminates legislative information. Holds an annual conference. Publications: *Central Lines*, quarterly newsletter; *Neonatal Network*, journal, 8 issues/year.

National Association of Orthopaedic Nurses (NAON)
  E. Holly Ave., Box 56
  Pitman, NJ 08071-0056
  609-256-2310, fax: 609-589-7463
  Dues: $60/year
Enhances personal and professional growth of orthopedic nurses through continuing education programs. Sponsors workshops, maintains a speakers' bureau, offers research grants. Runs an annual congress. Publications: *News*, bimonthly; *Orthopaedic Nursing*, bimonthly journal.

National Association of Vascular Access Nurses (NAVAN)
P.O. Box 52883
Irvine, CA 92619
500-442-4455, 714-442-1960, fax: 714-442-1590
Dues: $60/year

A multidisciplinary organization of health care professionals interested in advancing the practice of vascular access management. Offers continuing education courses, certification courses, local NAVAN networks, and regional meetings. Runs an annual educational convention. Publications: *Journal of Vascular Access,* quarterly, included with membership dues.

National Certification Corporation for the Obstetric,
Gynecologic, and Neonatal Nursing Specialties (NCC)
645 N. Michigan Ave., Suite 900
Chicago, IL 60611
800-367-5613, 312-951-0207

Promotes quality nursing care by encouraging nurses to demonstrate special knowledge by participating in a voluntary national certification program for ob/gyn nurse practitioners, inpatient obstetric nurses, neonatal intensive care nurses, low-risk neonatal nurses, reproductive endocrinology/infertility nurses, ambulatory women's health care nurses, high-risk obstetric nurses, and maternal newborn nurses. Holds an annual meeting. Publications: *NCC News,* periodic.

National Flight Nurses Association (NFNA)
c/o Steve Lieber
216 Higgins Rd.
Park Ridge, IL 60068
847-698-1733, fax: 847-698-9406
Dues: $65/year

Holds an annual conference in conjunction with Association of Air Medical Services, National Flight Paramedics Association, and Nation EMS Pilots Association; always held mid-year. Publications: *Across the Board*, bimonthly newsletter; *Journal of Air Medical Transport*, monthly.

Oncology Nursing Society (ONS)
    501 Holiday Dr.
    Pittsburgh, PA 15220
    412-921-7373, fax: 412-921-6565
    e-mail: member@ons.org
    Dues: $71/year
Seeks to promote high professional standards in oncology nursing; provide a network for the exchange of information, resources, and peer support; encourage nurses to specialize in oncology; promote and develop educational programs in oncology nursing; identify, encourage, and foster nursing research in improving the quality of patient care. Compiles statistics. Maintains speakers' bureau. Holds annual institute, always in the fall, and an annual congress.

Respiratory Nursing Society (RNS)
    437 Twin Bay Dr.
    Pensacola, FL 32534-1350
    904-474-8869, fax: 904-484-8762
    Dues: $75/year
Fosters the personal and professional development of respiratory nurses, and quality care of their clients. Provides educational opportunities and promotes research in the field. Publications: *Perspectives in Respiratory Nursing*, quarterly newsletter.

Society of Otorhinolaryngology & Head/Neck Nurses (SOHN)
116 Canal St., Suite A
New Smyrna Beach, FL 32168
904-428-1695, fax: 904-423-7566
Seeks to promote awareness of professional techniques and new developments in the field; enhance professional standards; create a channel for the exchange of ideas, concerns, and information; and develop interaction with similar groups. Offers programs and seminars approved for continuing education credits. Holds annual congress. Publications: *ORL-Head and Neck Nursing,* quarterly, included in membership dues, $30/year for non-members; *Society of Otorhinolaryngology and Head-Neck Nurses —Update,* quarterly newsletter, included in membership dues.

Society of Trauma Nurses (STN)
1211 Locust St.
Philadelphia, PA 19107
800-237-6966, 215-545-5687, fax: 215-545-8107
Dues: $50/year
Seeks to communicate trauma nursing information and recognize excellence and innovation in trauma nursing. Addresses legislative issues and assists in the development of standards. Publications: *Journal of Trauma Nursing,* quarterly, included in membership dues, $42/year for non-members.

Society for Vascular Nursing (SVN)
437 Twin Bay Dr.
Pensacola, FL 32534-1350
888-536-4786, fax: 904-484-8762
Dues: $75/year
Seeks to educate public about prevention of peripheral vascular disease, provides educational programs, conducts research. Operates speakers' bureau. Holds annual symposium every May or June. Publications: *Journal of Vascular Nursing,* quarterly, included in membership dues; *SVN.prn,* newsletter.

▲ Long-term care organizations

American Association for Continuity of Care (AACC)
638 Prospect Ave.
Hartford, CT 06105-4250
860-586-7525, fax: 860-586-7550

For health care professionals involved in discharge planning, social work, hospital administration, home care, long-term care, home health agencies, and continuity of care. Maintains speakers' bureau. Holds an annual conference. Publications: *Access*, 4 issues/year, included in membership dues; *IMPAACT*, bimonthly bulletin, included in membership dues.

American Health Care Association (AHCA)
1201 L St. NW
Washington, D.C. 20005
202-842-4444, fax: 202-842-3860

Promotes standards for professionals in long-term health care delivery, and quality care for patients and residents in a safe environment. Holds an annual conference. Publications: *AHCA Notes*, monthly newsletter, included in membership dues; *Provider: For Long-Term Care Professionals*, monthly magazine, included in membership, $48/year for non-members.

▲ Managed care/QA/risk management organizations

American Association of Managed Care Nurses (AAMCN)
P.O. Box 4975
Glen Ellen, VA 23058-4975
804-747-9698, fax: 804-747-5316
Dues: $95/year

Seeks to enhance the abilities of managed health care professionals through education, networking, and legislative lobbying. Conducts educational programs, and maintains speakers' bureau. Sponsors regional meetings for utilization management and quality assurance issues three times per year. Publications: *Nurses' Notes*, quarterly newsletter, included in membership dues.

American Society for Healthcare Risk Management (ASHRM)
American Hospital Association
One N. Franklin
Chicago, IL 60606
312-422-3980, fax: 312-422-4580

Purposes are to promote professional development of hospital risk managers, provide educational resources and programs on hospital risk management, and address risk management issues affecting the health care industry. Holds annual meeting. Publications: *Journal of Healthcare Risk Management*, quarterly, included in membership dues.

National Association for Healthcare Quality (NAHQ)
4700 W. Lake Ave.
Glenview, IL 60025-1485
847-375-4700, fax: 847-875-4777
Dues: $100

Objectives are to: encourage, develop, and provide continuing education for all persons involved in health care quality; give patients primary consideration in all actions affecting their health and welfare; promote the sharing of knowledge and encourage a high degree of professional ethics in health care. Offers accredited certification in the field of health care quality, utilization, and risk management. Conducts educational seminars and conferences. Holds NAHQ Annual Educational Conference. Publications: *Journal for Healthcare Quality*, bimonthly, $100/year; *NAHQ News*, quarterly newsletter.

Professional Standards Review Council of America (PSRCA)
200 Madison Ave., Suite 1910
New York, NY 10016
212-686-9147, fax: 212-779-9307

Monitors the quality, appropriateness, and cost of health care received by patients in hospitals, ambulatory clinics, nursing facilities, and physician's offices. Holds quarterly conferences and seminars. Publications: *Informational Health Care Bulletin*, periodic.

Quality Review Associates
    11818 Gateway Blvd. #7
    Los Angeles, CA 90064
    800-562-2160
Offers home-study course for nurses interested in the quality review arena.

▲ Occupational health organizations

American Association of Occupational Health Nurses (AAOHN)
    50 Lenox Pointe
    Atlanta, GA 30324-3176
    404-262-1162, fax: 404-262-1165
Promotes and sets standards for nurses employed by business and industrial firms. Provides continuing education, maintains governmental affairs program, and offers placement service. Sponsors the annual American Occupational Health Conference. Publications: *AAOHN Journal*, monthly; *AAOHN News*, monthly newsletter.

American Board for Occupational Health Nurses (ABOHN)
    9944 S. Roberts Rd., Suite 205
    Palos Hills, IL 60465-1555
    630-789-5799, fax: 630-789-8901
Establishes standards and confers initial and ongoing certification in occupational health nursing. Conducts annual certification examination. Publications: *The COHN Report*, semiannual newsletter; *Reference Guide for Examination Preparation*.

▲ *Outpatient nursing organizations*

American Academy of Ambulatory Care Nursing (AAACN)
    East Holly Ave., Box 56
    Pitman, NJ 08071-0056
    609-256-2350, fax: 609-589-7463
    Dues: $120/year

For nurses with administrative/management responsibilities in ambulatory care. Offers programs to enhance leadership and supervisory skills and improve members' abilities to influence organizational decisions. Ask about their special interest group (SIG) on telephone triage or telephone nursing services. Provides workshops, continuing education, and in-service educational programs. Annual conference, always in March. Publications: *Ambulatory Care Nursing Administration and Practice Standards*, $30 for members, $50 for non-members; *Dermatology Nursing*, journal; *MedSurg Nursing*, journal; *Nursing Economics*, bimonthly journal; *Pediatric Nursing*, journal; *Viewpoint*, bimonthly newsletter, included with membership dues.

American Association of Office Nurses
    109 Kenderkamack Rd.
    Montvale, NJ 07645
    201-391-2600, fax: 201-573-8543
    Dues: $35/year

Promotes improvement of the image of the office nurse. Encourages professional growth and development, and facilitates exchange of information among members. Provides continuing education opportunities. Sponsors an annual meeting and convention. Publications: *NEON*, quarterly newsletter.

American Psychiatric Nurses Association (APNA)
    c/o Carolyn Freeland
    1200 19th St. NW, Suite 300
    Washington, D.C. 20036
    202-857-1133, fax: 202-223-4579

e-mail: karie_noelle@sba.com

Dues: $100/year

Works to improve patient care by fostering clinical research and encouraging community involvement. Facilitates continuing education and professional development of members. Holds annual conference, always in October. Publications: *APNA News*, bimonthly newsletter; *Journal of the American Psychiatric Nurses Association*, bimonthly.

American Society of Ophthalmic Registered Nurses (ASORN)

P.O. Box 193030

San Francisco, CA 94119

415-561-8513, fax: 415-561-8575

e-mail: sarah_smith@uiowa.edu

Dues: $65/year

Promotes excellence in ophthalmic nursing. Facilitates continuing education through the study, discussion, and exchange of knowledge, experience, and ideas in the field. Conducts educational programs. Holds an annual conference. Publications: *Insight, The Journal of the American Society of Ophthalmic Registered Nurses*, quarterly, included in membership dues, $35/year for non-members.

American Society for Peri-Anesthesia Nurses

6900 Grove Rd.

Thorofare, NJ 08086

609-845-5557, fax: 609-848-1881

e-mail: aspan@slackinc.com

Serves nurses practicing in ambulatory surgery, pre-anesthesia and post-anesthesia care. Promotes quality and cost-effective care for patients, their families, and the community through public education, research, and standards of practice. Holds an annual conference, regional workshops, seminars, independent study, and certification courses. Publications: *Journal of Peri-Anesthesia Nursing; Breathline*, newsletter.

American Society of Plastic and Reconstructive Surgical Nurses (ASPRSN)

> E. Holly Ave., Box 56
> Pitman, NJ 08071
> 609-256-2340, fax: 609-589-7463

Objectives are to enhance leadership qualities of nurses in the field of plastic surgery; increase the skills, knowledge, and understanding of personnel in plastic surgery through continuing education; encourage participation and interest in professional organizations; and cooperate with others in the profession. Holds an annual meeting. Publications: *ASPRS News*, bimonthly newsletter, included in membership dues; *Plastic Surgical Nursing*, quarterly journal.

Association of Child and Adolescent Psychiatric Nurses (ACAPN)

> 1211 Locust St.
> Philadelphia, PA 19107
> 800-826-2950, 215-545-2843, fax: 215-545-8107
> Dues: $90/year, $55/year for students.

Works to promote mental health of infants, children, adolescents, and their families through clinical practice, public policy, and research. Holds an annual conference, usually in the fall. Publications: *ACAPN News*, newsletter, 3 issues/year, included in membership dues, $20 for non-members; *Journal of Child & Adolescent Psychiatric Nursing*, quarterly, included in membership dues, $43/year for non-members.

Dermatology Nurses' Association (DNA)

> E. Holly Ave. Box 56
> Pitman, NJ 08071
> 609-256-2330, fax: 609-589-7463

Addresses professional issues involving dermatology nurses, develops standards of care, facilitates communication and interdisciplinary cooperation among members. Conducts educational meetings. Holds an annual conference every summer. Publications: Newsletter, bimonthly.

International TeleNurses Association (ITA)
    10711 Bexley Drive
    Houston, TX 77099
    e-mail: ita96@aol.com *or:* gsuhr@msmail.his.tch.tmc.edu
Promotes and supports nursing involvement in telehealth. Telehealth includes distant patient and professional consultations and education, telephone triage, teleradiology, and other applications. Promotes standards within telehealth which provide and promote quality patient care.

National Consortium of Chemical Dependency Nurses (NCCDN)
    1720 Willow Creek Cir., Suite 519
    Eugene, OR 97402
    800-87-NCCDN, 503-485-4421, fax: 503-485-7372
    Dues: $50/year
Goals are to increase the effectiveness of nursing services for chemical dependency, and establish a professional standard in chemical dependency nursing through a system of competency-based testing and programs of professional development and certification. Offers certification exam for nurses with 4,000 hours of experience in the previous five years and 30 hours of chemical dependency coursework. Conducts educational programs. Maintains speakers' bureau. Holds an annual CD Nurse Conference and meeting. Publications: *CD Nurse Briefing*, quarterly newsletter.

National Nurses Society on Addictions (NNSA)
    4101 Lake Boone Trail, Suite 201
    Raleigh, NC 27607
    919-783-5871, fax: 919-787-4916
    Dues: $80/year

Fosters continuing education and development of skills among nurses involved in the field. Works to enhance the professional image of addictions nurses. Provides certification program. Holds an annual conference. Publications: *Perspectives on Addictions Nursing,* quarterly newsletter, $20/year for non-members.

▲ Professional nursing organizations

American Academy of Nurse Practitioners (AANP)
    LBJ Building
    P.O. Box 12846, Capital Station
    Austin, TX 78711
    512-442-4262, fax: 512-442-6469
Promotes high standards of health care delivered by nurse practitioners. Supports continuing education programs, encourages research in the field, and compiles statistics. Holds an annual continuing education conference. Publications: *Academy Update,* monthly newsletter; *Journal of the American Academy of Nurse Practitioners,* quarterly (focuses on clinical practice, management, and education), available online.

American College of Nurse Midwives (ACNM)
    818 Connecticut Ave. NW #900
    Washington, D.C. 20006
    202-728-9860, fax: 202-728-9897
Plans and develops educational programs, conducts research and continuing education workshops, sponsors research, compiles statistics, maintains speakers' bureau and archives, and offers placement service to nurse midwives. Holds an annual conference. Publications: *Journal of Nurse-Midwifery,* bimonthly, included in membership dues, $48/year for non-members; *Quickening,* bimonthly newsletter, included in membership dues.

American Licensed Practical Nurses Association (ALPNA)
1090 Vermont Ave. NW, Suite 1200
Washington, D.C. 20005
202-682-9000, fax: 202-298-6686

Promotes the practical nursing profession, lobbies on issues that may have an impact on LPNs, conducts continuing education classes, and facilitates discussion of issues affecting the nursing and health professions. Holds annual conference every August.

American Nurses Association (ANA)
600 Maryland Ave. SW, Suite 100W
Washington, D.C. 20024-2571
202-651-7000, fax: 202-651-7001
e-mail: chelmlin@ana.org

Represents registered nurses, sponsors numerous committees and councils. Sponsors biennial meeting and the annual House of Delegates meeting. Publications: *The American Journal of Nursing*, monthly magazine, $22.97/year, call 800-CALL-AJN; *The American Nurse*, newspaper, includes employment listings, included with membership dues, $20/year for non-members, $10/year for students; *Facts About Nursing*, semiannual; *Proceedings of the House of Delegates*, periodic.

American Nurses' Foundation (ANF)
600 Maryland Ave. SW, Suite 100W
Washington, D.C. 20024-2571
202-651-7227, fax: 202-651-7001

Provides continuing education opportunities; sponsors demonstration projects, research, and other programs for nurses to enhance health care delivery. Board meeting three times/year.

International Council of Nurses
   3 Place Jean Marteau
   1201 Geneva
   Switzerland

National Association of Registered Nurses (NARN)
   11508 Allecingie Pkwy., Suite C
   Richmond, VA   23235
   804-794-6513, fax: 804-379-7698
   Dues: $10/year
Seeks to offer nurses the opportunity to plan and create a finan-
cially sound future through financial management programs.
Provides financial products, consultation and services including
IRAs, full investment services, and group life insurance. Con-
ducts educational programs.

National Association of School Nurses (NASN)
   P.O. Box 1300
   Scarborough, ME   04070-1300
   207-883-2117, fax: 207-883-2683
   e-mail: NASN@aol.com
   Dues: $60/year
Objectives are to provide national leadership in the promotion
of health services for schoolchildren, promote school health interests to the nursing/health community and the public, and
monitor legislation pertaining to school nursing. Provides continuing education programs. Has established workshops and
grants for study of child and drug abuse, the female body, and
skin care. Holds an annual conference, usually the last weekend in June. Publications: *Journal of School Nursing*, quarterly
magazine; *NASNewsletter*, quarterly, included in membership
dues.

National Federation of Licensed Practical Nurses (NFLPN)
1418 Aversboro Rd.
Garner, NC 27529-4547
919-779-0046, fax: 919-779-5642

Aims to preserve and foster the ideal of comprehensive nursing care for the ill and aged, improve standards of practice, secure recognition and effective utilization of LPNs, and further continued improvement in the education of LPNs. Maintains loan program. Holds an annual convention. Publications: *Licensed Practical Nurse*, quarterly journal.

National Federation for Specialty Nursing Organizations (NFSNO)
E. Holly Ave., Box 56
Pitman, NJ 08071
609-256-2333, fax: 609-589-7463

Provides a forum for discussion of issues of mutual concern to members, attempts to gain more input in establishing of nursing standards. Holds an annual meeting every fourth weekend in July. Publications: *NFSNO Focus on the Federation*, quarterly newsletter.

National League for Nursing (NLN)
350 Hudson St.
New York, NY 10014
800-669-1656, 212-989-9393, fax: 212-989-3710
e-mail: nlninform@nln.org

Works to assess nursing needs, improve organized nursing services and nursing education, and foster collaboration between nursing and other health and community services. Provides tests used select applicants to schools of nursing, and prepares tests for evaluating nursing student progress and nursing service tests. Nationally accredits nursing education programs and community health agencies. Collects and disseminates data on nursing services and education. Ask for information/video on "How to start a Nursing Center." Holds a biennial conference. Publications: *NLN Newsletter*, periodic; *Nursing and Health Care*, journal, 10 issues/year; *Nursing Data Review*, annual; *Nursing Student Census*, annual.

National Organization for Associate Degree Nursing (NOADN)
    11250 Roger Bacon Dr., Suite 8
    Reston, VA 20190
    703-437-4377, fax: 703-435-4390
Represents and advances the status of associate degree nursing education and practice. Provides networking among members to facilitate the exchange of legislative information and support. Holds an annual convention. Publications: Quarterly newsletter.

National Student Nurses' Association
    555 West 57th St., Suite 1327
    New York, NY 10019
    212-581-2211, fax: 212-581-2368
Provides information and support to nursing students nationwide. Publications available for members.

World Health Organization
    Avenue Appia 1211
    Geneva 27
    Switzerland

▲ *Rehabilitation/cardiac rehab organizations*

American Association of Cardiovascular and Pulmonary
Rehabilitation (AACVPR)
   7611 Elmwood Ave., Suite 201
   Middleton, WI 53562
   608-831-6989, fax: 608-831-5122
Fosters the improvement of clinical practice in CVPR, promotes
scientific CVPR research, and seeks the advancement of CVPR
education for health care professionals and the public. Holds an
annual conference. Publications: *Journal of Cardiopulmonary
Rehabilitation*, bimonthly, included in membership dues, $120/
year for non-members.

Association of Rehabilitation Nurses (ARN)
   4700 W. Lake Ave.
   Glenview, IL 60025-1485
   800-229-7530, 847-375-4710, fax: 847-375-4777
   Dues: $95/year
Works to advance the quality of rehabilitation nursing practice
through educational opportunities and facilitate the exchange
of ideas. Holds an annual conference. Publications: *Application
of Rehabilitation Concepts to Nursing Practice: Self-Study*, audio-
tapes; *ARN Newsletter*, 10 issues/year; *Rehabilitation Nursing
Journal*, bimonthly; *Rehabilitation Nursing Research*, quarterly,
$35/year for members, $65/year for non-members; *Rehabilitation
Nursing: Scope of Practice*.

▲ Special interest organizations

American Assembly for Men in Nursing (AAMN)
437 Twin Bay Dr.
Pensacola, FL 32534-1350
904-474-0144, fax: 904-484-8762
e-mail: aamn@aol.com

Works to help eliminate prejudice in nursing, interest men in the profession, encourage education, and promote further professional growth. Conducts educational programs. Sponsors an annual conference. Publications: *Interaction*, quarterly newsletter, included in membership dues.

Lesbian and Gay Nurses' Alliance
801 E. Harrison Suite 105
Seattle, WA 98102

National Association of Hispanic Nurses (NAHN)
1501 16th St. NW
Washington, D.C. 20036
202-387-2477, fax: 202-797-4353
Dues: $50/year

Serves the nursing and health care delivery needs of the Hispanic community and the professional needs of Hispanic nurses. Holds annual convention. Publications: *Hispanic Nurse*, quarterly, $15/year.

National Black Nurses Association (NBNA)
1511 K St. NW, Suite 415
Washington, D.C. 20005
202-393-6870, fax: 202-347-3808

Functions as a professional support group and an advocacy group for the black community and its health care. Recruits and assists blacks interested in pursuing nursing as a career. Presents scholarships to student nurses, compiles statistics, maintains biographical archives and charitable program. Holds an annual conference. Publications: *Journal of Black Nurses Association*, semi-annual, included in membership dues; *NBNA Newsletter*, quarterly, included in membership dues.

Nurses Organization of Veterans Affairs (NOVA)
   1726 M. St. NW, Suite 1101
   Washington, D.C. 20036
   202-296-0888, fax: 202-833-1577
   Dues: $70/year
Objective is to provide VA nurses with the opportunity to preserve and improve quality care and professionalism through legislative influence. Conducts competitions, seminars, and educational programs. Holds an annual conference. Publications: *News from NOVA*, quarterly newsletter, $40/year for nonmembers.

STATE NURSING ASSOCIATIONS

Alabama Nurses' Association
360 N. Hull St.
Montgomery, AL 36104
334-262-8321, fax: 334-262-8578

Alaska Nurses' Association
237 E. 3rd Ave., #3
Anchorage, AK 99501
907-274-0827, fax: 907-272-0292

Arizona Nurses' Association
1850 E. Southern, Suite #1
Tempe, AZ 85282
602-831-0404, fax: 602-839-4780

California Nurses' Association
1145 Market St., Suite 1100
San Francisco, CA 94103
415-864-4141, fax: 415-863-1325

Colorado Nurses' Association
5453 East Evans Place
Denver, CO 80222
303-757-7484, fax: 303-757-2679

Connecticut Nurses' Association
377 Research Pkwy.
Meridian, CT 06450
203-238-1207, fax: 203-238-3437

Delaware Nurses' Association
2634 Capitol Trail, Suite A
Newark, DE 19711
302-368-2333, fax: 302-366-1775

District of Columbia Nurses' Association
5100 Wisconsin Ave. NW, Suite 306
Washington, D.C. 20016
202-244-2705, fax: 202-362-8285

Florida Nurses' Association
P.O. Box 536985
Orlando, FL 32853-6985
407-896-3261, fax: 407-896-9042

Georgia Nurses' Association
1362 W. Peachtree St. NW
Atlanta, GA 30309
404-876-4624, fax: 404-876-4621

Hawaii Nurses' Association
677 Alamoana Blvd., Suite 301
Honolulu, HI 96813
808-531-1628, fax: 808-524-2760

Idaho Nurses' Association
200 N. 4th, Suite 20
Boise, ID 83702
208-345-0500, fax: 208-385-0166

Illinois Nurses' Association
300 S. Wacker Dr., Suite 2200
Chicago, IL 60606
312-360-2300, 312-360-9380

Indiana Nurses' Association
2915 N. High School Rd.
Indianapolis, IN 46224
317-299-4575, fax: 317-297-3525

Iowa Nurses' Association
Iowa Department of Health
321 E. 12th St. – Lucas Building
Des Moines, IA 50319
515-281-3255, fax: 515-281-3121

Kansas Nurses' Association
700 SW Jackson, Suite 601
Topeka, KS 66603
913-233-8638, fax: 913-233-5222

Kentucky Nurses' Association
P.O. Box 2616
Louisville, KY 40201
502-637-2546, fax: 502-637-8236

Louisiana Nurses' Association
712 Trans Continental Dr.
Metarie, LA 70001
504-889-1030, fax: 504-888-1158

Maine Nurses' Association
P.O. Box 2240
Augusta, ME 04338-2240
207-622-1057, fax: 207-623-4072

Maryland Nurses' Association
849 International Dr., Suite 255
Linthicum, MD 21090
410-859-3000, fax: 410-859-3001

Massachusetts Nurses' Association
340 Turnpike St.
Canton, MA 02021
617-821-4625, fax: 617-821-4445

Michigan Nurses' Association
2310 Jolly Oak Rd.
Okemos, MI 48864
517-349-5640, fax: 517-349-5818

Minnesota Nurses' Association
1295 Bandana Blvd. N., Suite 140
St. Paul, MN 55108
612-646-4807, fax: 612-647-5301

Mississippi Nurses' Association
135 Bounds St.
Jackson, MS 39206
601-982-9182, fax: 601-982-9183

Missouri Nurses' Association
P.O. Box 105228
Jefferson City, MO 65110
573-636-4623, fax: 573-636-9576

Montana Nurses' Association
P.O. Box 5718
Helena, MT 59604
406-442-6710, fax: 406-442-1841

Nebraska Nurses' Association
1430 South St., Suite 202
Lincoln, NE 68502
402-475-3859, fax: 402-475-3961

Nevada Nurses' Association
P.O. Box 2777
Reno, NV 89505
702-323-1661, fax: 702-323-0648

New Hampshire Nurses' Association
48 West St.
Concord, NH 03301-3595
603-225-3783, fax: 603-228-6672

New Jersey Nurses' Association
1479 Pennington Rd.
Trenton, NJ 08618
609-392-4884, fax: 609-883-5343

New Mexico Nurses' Association
909 Virginia Ave. NE
Albuquerque, NM 87108
505-268-7744, fax: 505-268-7711

New York Nurses' Association
46 Cornell Rd.
Latham, NY 12110
518-782-9400, fax: 518-782-9530

North Carolina Nurses' Association
P.O. Box 12025
Raleigh, NC 27605
919-821-4250, fax: 919-829-5807

North Dakota Nurses' Association
549 Airport Rd.
Bismarck, ND 58504-6107
701-223-1385, fax: 701-223-0575

Ohio Nurses' Association
4000 E. Main St.
Columbus, OH 43213
614-237-5414, fax: 614-237-6074

Oklahoma Nurses' Association
6414 N. Santa Fe, #A
Oklahoma City, OK 73116-9114
405-840-3476, fax: 405-840-3013

Oregon Nurses' Association
9600 SW Oak St., Suite 550
Portland, OR 97223
503-293-0011, fax: 503-293-0013

Pennsylvania Nurses' Association
P.O. Box 68525
Harrisburg, PA 17106-8525
717-657-1222, fax: 717-657-3796

Rhode Island Nurses' Association
550 S. Water St.
Providence, RI 02903
401-421-9703, fax: 401-421-6793

South Carolina Nurses' Association
1821 Gadsden St.
Columbia, SC 29201
803-252-4781, fax: 803-779-3870

South Dakota Nurses' Association
1505 S. Minnesota, Suite 3
Sioux Falls, SD 57105
605-338-1401

Tennessee Nurses' Association
545 Mainstream Dr., Suite 405
Nashville, TN 37228
615-254-0350, fax: 615-254-0303

Texas Nurses' Association
7600 Burnet Rd., Suite 440
Austin, TX 78757
512-452-0645, fax: 512-452-0648

Utah Nurses' Association
455 East 400 South, Suite 50
Salt Lake City, UT 84111
801-322-3439, fax: 801-322-3430

Vermont Nurses' Association
Champlain Mill #26
1 Main St.
Winooski, VT 05404
802-655-7123, fax: 802-655-7187

Virginia Nurses' Association
7113 Three Chomp Rd., Suite 204
Richmond, VA 23226
804-282-1808, fax: 804-282-4916

Washington Nurses' Association
2505 2nd Ave., Suite 500
Seattle, WA 98121
206-443-9762, fax: 206-728-2074

West Virginia Nurses' Association
P.O. Box 1946
Charleston, WV 25327
304-342-1169, fax: 304-342-6973

Wisconsin Nurses' Association
6117 Monona Dr.
Madison, WI 53716
608-221-0383, fax: 608-221-2788

Wyoming Nurses Association
1603 Capitol Ave., Suite 305
Cheyenne, WY 82001
307-635-3955, fax: 307-635-2173

ONLINE RESOURCES

There are a *tremendous* number of resources available for nurses online. While I cannot even begin to list them all here, I've included some of my favorite "entry points" into the Internet world of nursing and a variety of options for the online nurse. Happy surfing!

▲ *Web pages*

Nurseweek.com/ (general nursing information and *lots* of links)

Wholenurse.com/ (general nursing information and *lots* of links)

NursingNet.org/ (general nursing information, student nurse information)

AORN.org/ (Association of Operating Room Nurses)

Rehabnurse.org/ (Association of Rehab Nurses)

ENA.org/ (Emergency Nurses' Association)

Ajn.org/ajnnet/hrsorgs/nann/ (National Association of Neonatal Nurses)

vrmedia.com/nurses/ (School Nurses)

ONS.org/ (Oncology Nurses Society)

Ahna.org/ (Holistic Nursing Association)

ana.org/ojin/ojinhome.htm (online journal of issues in nursing)

▲ *Electronic mailing lists*

An electronic mailing list contains the e-mail address of anyone who subscribes to the mailing list. When someone sends a message to the mailing list address, the message is copied and sent to the e-mail address of everyone on the mailing list. By subscribing to a healthcare mailing list, you can read and participate in interesting discussions. But beware: When you subscribe to a mailing list, you can receive up to 100 messages per day directly to your e-mail address. Be sure you save the instructions from your list server about how to "unsubscribe" to the mailing list.

To subscribe to an e-mail list, send an e-mail message to the address, type "SUBSCRIBE" on the subject line, and put the "subscribe" command followed by yourfirstname and yourlastname (put a space only *between* your first and last name) in the body of the message. For example, for the Nursing Educators discussion group:

listserv@ulkyvm.louisville.edu (the address)

SUBSCRIBE (subject line)

subscribe NRSINGED Zardoya Eagles (goes in the body
    of the message)

The address and message *must* be exact, or the listserve will not accept your subscription.

This is a sampling of the many e-mail lists available. For a more complete selection, search for *lists of list servers* online.

Culture and Nursing: majordomo@itssrv1.ucsf.edu
subscribe CULTURE-AND-NURSING your e-mail address

Flight Nurses: listserv@rotor.com
subscribe FLIGHTMED yourfirstname yourlastname

Geriatric Nurses: listserv@ubvm.bitnet
subscribe GERINET yourfirstname yourlastname

Home Health Nurses: listserv@usa.net
subscribe HOMEHLTH yourfirstname yourlastname

Home Care and Hospice Nurses:
    majordomo@po.cwru.edu
subscribe HCARENURS yourfirstname yourlastname

International TeleNurses Association (ITA):
    listserv@listserv.bcm.tmc.edu
subscribe ITNA yourfirstname yourlastname

IV Therapy: ivtherapy-l@netcom.com
    or ivtherapy-l-request@netcom.com
subscribe ivtherapy@netcom.com yourfirstname
    yourlastname

Midwife: midwife-request@asv.warwick.ac.uk
subscribe yourfirstname yourlastname

Nurse Faculty: carenetl@humber.bitnet
subscribe CARENETL yourfirstname yourlastname

Nurse Researcher: listserve@kentvm.kent.edu
    or listserv@kentvm
sub NurseRes yourfirstname yourlastname

Nurse Practitioner: npinfo@npl.com
subscribe yourfirstname yourlastname

Nursing Administration, Practice, Education and Research:
    listserv@vm.utcc.utoronto.ca
Subscribe nursenet yourfirstname yourlastname

Nursing Informatics: listproc@lists.umass.edu
sub nrsing-l yourfirstname yourlastname

Nursing Educators discussion group:
    listserv@ulkyvm.louisville.edu
sub NRSINGED yourfirstname yourlastname

Nursing Students: listserv@abvm.cc.buffalo.edu
    or listserv@ubvm.bitnet
subscribe snurse-l yourfirstname yourlastname

Occupational Therapy Nurses: mailserv@ac.dal.ca
subscribe Occup-ther yourfirstname yourlastname

Ophthalmic Nurses: maiser@mailgw.ornet.med.umich.edu
subscribe yourfirstname yourlastname

Perinatal Nursing: pnatalmrn@ubvm.bitnet
subscribe PNATALRN yourfirstname yourlastname

Professional Nursing issues: listserv@vm.utcc.utoronto.ca
subscribe NurseNet yourfirstname yourlastname

Psychiatric Nurses: mailbase@mailbase.ac.uk
join psychiatric-nursing yourfirstname yourlastname

Quality Practices: majordomo@quality.org
subscribe QP-health

School Nurses: schlrn-l@ubvm.bitnet
subscribe SCHLRN-L yourfirstname yourlastname

Index

Sovereignty Press is a publishing company committed to producing and distributing products that contribute to individual growth, development, and personal empowerment. We specialize in publications for nurses and other health care professionals that address past and present trends, personal and professional evolution, and the growth of professional stature and esteem.

We believe that individual growth and development (or sovereignty) is a prerequisite to the evolution of humanity, and that each person who undergoes this personal journey of growth can then step forward and make their own unique contribution to the world—thereby contributing to the evolution of all.

If you have an interest in publishing *your* great contribution, send inquiries to:

Sovereignty Press
1241 Johnson Avenue, #353
San Luis Obispo, CA 93401